ABDOMINAL ACCESS IN OPEN AND LAPAROSCOPIC SURGERY

ABDOMINAL ACCESS IN OPEN AND LAPAROSCOPIC SURGERY

EDITED BY

EDMUND K. M. TSOI, M.D.
CLAUDE H. ORGAN, Jr., M.D.
University of California—Davis, East Bay
Department of Surgery

NEW ENGLAND INSTITUTE
OF TECHNOLOGY
LEARNING RESOURCES CENTER

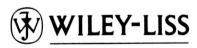

WILEY-LISS

A JOHN WILEY & SONS, INC., PUBLICATION
New York • Chichester • Brisbane • Toronto • Singapore

2/99

33983738

Library of Congress Cataloging-in-Publication Data:
Abdominal access in open and laparoscopic surgery / editors, Edmund
  K. M. Tsoi, Claude H. Organ, Jr.
      p. cm.
    Includes bibliographical references and index.
    ISBN 0-471-13352-3 (cloth : alk. paper)
    1. Abdomen—Endoscopic surgery.   2. Cutdown (Surgery)
3. Pneumoperitoneum, Artificial.   I. Tsoi, Edmund K. M.
II. Organ, Claude H. Jr., 1928–   .
    [DNLM: 1. Surgery, Laparoscopic—methods.   2. Pneumoperitoneum,
Artificial—methods.   3. Nitrous Oxide—administration & dosage.
WO 500 A135 1996]
RD540.A17   1996
617.5′5059—dc20   95-49690

Printed in the United States of America

10 9 8 7 6 5 4 3 2 1

To students of surgery, old and young
whose creative efforts continue to improve the quality of patient care

CONTRIBUTORS

David M. Brams, M.D. Assistant Clinical Professor of Surgery, University of California, Davis, East Bay Department of Surgery, Oakland, CA 94602

Albert K. Chin, M.D. Vice President of Research, Origin Medsystems, Inc., Menlo Park, CA

Lawrence J. Goldstein, M.D. Chief of Vascular Surgery, Alameda County Medical Center, Oakland, CA

Jay K. Harness, M.D. Professor of Surgery, University of California, Davis, East Bay Department of Surgery, Oakland, CA 94602

Vernon J. Henderson, M.D. Assistant Professor of Surgery, University of California, Davis, East Bay Department of Surgery, Oakland, CA 94602

Elsa R. Hirvela, M.D. Assistant Professor of Surgery, University of California, Davis, East Bay Department of Surgery, Oakland, CA 94602

Frederic H. Moll, M.D. Vice President and Medical Director, Origin Medsystems, Inc., Menlo Park, CA

Hideo Nagai, M.D. Associate Professor of Surgery, Jichi Medical School, Tochigi, Japan

Brian C. Organ, M.D. Assistant Clinical Professor of Surgery, Emory University, Atlanta, GA

Claude H. Organ, Jr., M.D. Professor and Chairman, University of California, Davis, East Bay Department of Surgery, Oakland, CA 94602

Gerald W. Peskin, M.D.   Clinical Professor of Surgery, University of California, Davis, East Bay Department of Surgery, Oakland, CA 94602

Edmund K. M. Tsoi, M.S., M.D.   Assistant Clinical Professor of Surgery, University of California, Davis, East Bay Department of Surgery, Oakland, CA 94602

Diana Vogt, M.D.   Chief Resident in Surgery, University of California, Davis, East Bay Department of Surgery, Oakland, CA 94602

Sunil K. Walia, M.D.   Surgical Resident, University of California, San Diego, CA

PREFACE

The introduction of minimally invasive surgery has blended basic concepts that have been operative in our field for many years with improved technology. We are currently functioning with the first generation of equipment not specially designed for minimally invasive surgery. If the past is any indication of the future, improvements in both instrumentation and videoscopy will expand minimally invasive surgery to include an even greater array of procedures.

Where the training of young surgeons and the introduction of new procedures overlap, we are professionally obligated to monitor both very carefully to assure that patients do not experience increased morbidity for the learning curve of either. It is our further mandate to accurately collect, analyze, and report the results of our studies for peer review. The surgical practices of today were dictated by the research of yesterday; tomorrow will be no different. It is axiomatic that there be continuing controlled clinical studies undertaken to validate new methods of treatment and to identify areas of morbidity and mortality. This is an exciting era of surgical history that permits us to combine the accumulated basic principles of the surgical sciences with recent technological advancements to improve our methods of diagnosis and expand management options for patients. These should be the abiding principles of the rapidly expanding new era in modern surgery.

CLAUDE H. ORGAN, JR.

ACKNOWLEDGMENTS

The editors are indebted to the professional efforts of Ms. Martha Steele and Ms. Margaret Kosiba in bringing this manuscript to completion. We are further indebted to Shawn H. Morton, Medical Editor at John Wiley & Sons, Inc., for his suggestions, encouragement, and support.

CONTENTS

OVERVIEW OF ABDOMINAL ACCESS

Edmund K. M. Tsoi, M.S., M.D.
Claude H. Organ, Jr., M.D.

I. INTRODUCTION

Access, exposure, and judgment are key elements in the design of a successful operation. In the past, making long incisions was the gold standard of gaining access into the abdominal and thoracic cavities. Since the introduction of videoscopic technology, long incisions have been replaced by trocars. In this chapter we will give an overview of three major methods of gaining access for abdominal surgery: (1) intraabdominal access, (2) intraluminal access, and (3) extraperitoneal access. Subsequent chapters will concentrate on various methods of open and laparoscopic surgery.

II. INTRAABDOMINAL ACCESS

Traditionally surgeons have gained access into the abdominal cavity via the anterior abdominal wall. In the age of minimally invasive surgery, incisions

Abdominal Access in Open and Laparoscopic Surgery
Edited by Edmund K. M. Tsoi and Claude H. Organ, Jr.
ISBN 0-471-13352-3 Copyright © 1996 by Wiley-Liss, Inc.

have been replaced by multiple trocar insertions and direct vision and tactile sensation by videoscopy. As more experience is gained, additional complicated procedures are being performed with the aid of the laparoscope combined with the technique of miniincision. In general, the appropriately placed access—trocar(s) and/or miniincision(s)—facilitate anatomical exposure and improve vision, minimizing postoperative complications.

Surgeons universally agree that adequate exposure is the most important technical aspect of an operation. In open procedures, exposure is best obtained by the assistant and an ever expanding traditional instrumentation. In conventional laparoscopic surgery, pneumoperitoneum aids the exposure by displacing abdominal contents and abdominal wall elevation. Specially designed laparoscopic retractors are useful in achieving needed exposure. These mechanical retractors are far from ideal. They are often difficult to employ or fail to adjust to the contour of the abdominal structures. A well-designed retractor is usually one that mimics those used in open surgery, including the hands of the assistants. Current instrumentation employed in videoscopic surgery should be considered a first-generation development. Technology is expected to develop, produce, and distribute a second generation of minimally invasive instruments more specifically designed to meet the needs for adequate surgical exposure.

In open surgery, a midline vertical or transverse incision enables the surgeon to perform almost any abdominal procedure. These incisions carry potential morbidity associated with pain and large scars. As a result, surgeons have used smaller incisions for organ-specific procedures when there is a high degree of certainty. For example, subcostal incisions are commonly used for splenectomy and cholecystectomy, and McBurney's or Rocky-Davis incisions for appendectomy. In those circumstances where a misdiagnosis is encountered, the surgeon must be knowledgeable as to how the incision can be extended. This requires a basic knowledge of the musculoaponeurotic structures of the anterior abdominal wall. A separate incision may be required if the surgeon needs better exposure.

In minimally invasive surgery, laparoscopy may facilitate the diagnosis of intraabdominal pathology. Most trocar placements in conventional laparoscopic surgery are located around the pathology, that is, the organ targeted for the operation. To remote the organ from the abdomen may necessitate miniincisions near the targeted structure to minimize air leak and to facilitate the extraction. Occasionally, a surgeon will encounter a situation where the procedure must be converted from a laparoscopic approach to open surgery. This decision is the earmark of a mature surgeon. Under these circumstances, an adequate midline or transverse incision to gain ample access to and exposure of the abdominal cavity is utilized.

III. INTRALUMINAL ACCESS

Besides incisions and trocars, another diagnostic and therapeutic method for gaining access to the abdominal structures is endoscopy. It was not utilized by many surgeons in the past because of lack of training or because they relegated their role to the gastroenterologist. With the development of the flexible video-endoscope, surgeons can easily perform diagnostic and therapeutic interventions via intraluminal access with minimal patient discomfort. Surgeons who perform their own endoscopies will likely have more insight into their patients' disease. Performing esophageal and colorectal surgery based upon the endoscopic findings of someone else is less than ideal and places the surgeon in a precarious position.

We now know that early gastrointestinal malignancy can be treated with endoscopic excision (Figure 1.1). Palliative treatment for advanced malignancy can also be performed with endoscopic techniques, for example, (1) balloon dilatation and/or intraluminal stenting for biliary or gastrointestinal malignant obstruction and (2) laser therapy for esophageal tumor. Benign diseases that have been successfully treated by endoscopic interventions include gastrointestinal hemorrhage, bile duct obstruction (secondary to stones or stricture), gastrointestinal obstruction resulting from acid or caustic substance ingestion, esophageal motility disorders (achalasia, diffuse esophageal spasm, scleroderma), peptic ulcer disease, gastroesophageal reflux, colonic volvulus (Figure 1.2), and pseudoobstruction (Ogilvie's syndrome). Foreign bodies in the gastrointestinal tract can frequently be removed using intraluminal endoscopy, thereby avoiding open surgery (Figure 1.3).

When combined with open or laparoscopic surgery, the fiber-optic endoscope can also facilitate the exposure of the operating field. One such application is the placement of a flexible sigmoidoscope in the rectum to transilluminate a Hartman's pouch during a colostomy take-down. This technique allows the surgeon to use the light as a guide with the endoscope in the bowel lumen as a handle for manipulation during dissection. Surgeons have used lap-

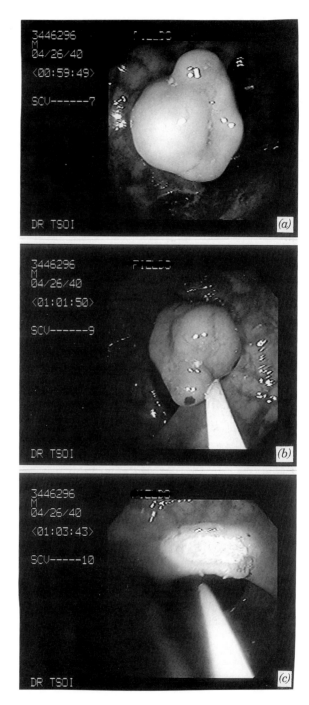

Figure 1.1. (*a*) Polyp identified during colonoscopy; (*b*) polypectomy with a snare; (*c*) cauterized mucosal surface after polypectomy. (See insert for color representation.)

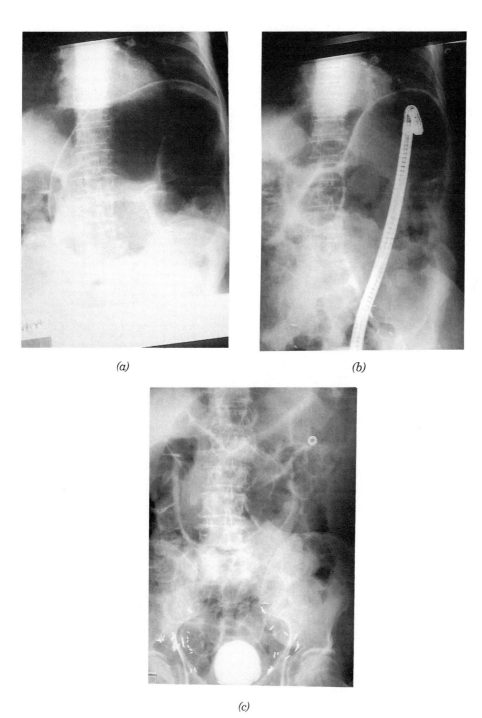

(a)

(b)

(c)

Figure 1.2. (a) Sigmoid volvulus seen on plain abdominal radiography; (b) reduction of volvulus with a flexible endoscope; (c) postreduction film. (See insert for color representation.)

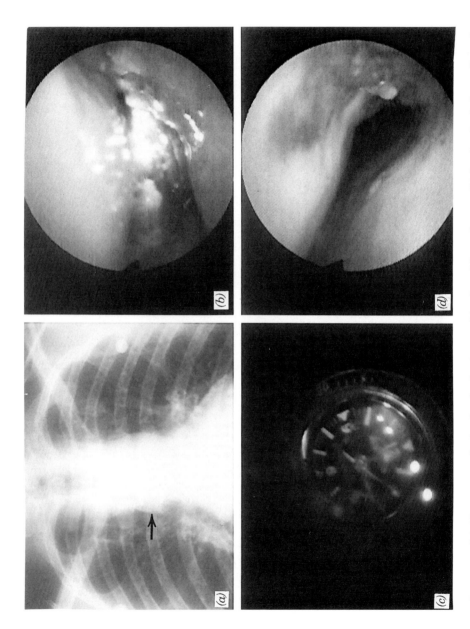

Figure 1.3. (*a*) Chest x-ray of a foreign body observed in the mid esophagus; (*b*) foreign body is confirmed by esophagoscopy; (*c*) the foreign body (a wrist watch) removed via esophagoscopy; (*d*) superficial mucosal ulceration after foreign body removal. (See insert for color representation.)

aroscopy to monitor colonoscopic polypectomy.[1] Others have used a flexible gastroscope to identify duodenal microgastrinomas. Payne and colleagues have used a flexible gastroscope to identify and monitor the laparoscopic removal of small gastric leiomyomas.[2] Another therapeutic use of the endoscope is to perform laparoscopic antegrade sphincterotomy in the management of choledocholithiasis.[3] This technique expands the ability of the surgeon to provide definitive management of both cholelithiasis and choledocholithiasis without additional preoperative endoscopic procedures.

The technique of intraluminal access that has replaced open surgery is the placement of gastric enteral access for nutritional support. In 1981, Gauderer and Ponsky used the fiber-optic endoscope to transilluminate the stomach for percutaneous endoscopic gastrostomy (PEG).[4] Another similar technique by Russell and associates has added to the progressively decreasing utilization of open gastrostomy.[5] Russell paved the way for further expansion of intraluminal access in laparoscopic surgery.

Recently, surgeons have investigated the use of the flexible gastroscope to inflate the stomach to expose an operating field in the excision of gastric cancer.[6] With this intraluminal technique, the stomach is first inflated with the help of a flexible gastroscope. The stomach is then transilluminated for the laparoscopic surgeon to place trocars directly through the abdominal wall into the stomach. Additional insufflation of the stomach can be achieved by connecting the gas port of the trocar to an insufflator. A rigid laparoscope is placed into the stomach via the trocar for intraluminal endoscopy. Once the lesion is identified, additional trocars can be placed into the stomach for surgical instruments (Figure 1.4). Filipi and associates have used the intraluminal approach to manage gastric bezoars.[7] In their technique, multiple percutaneous endoscopic gastrostomies were used as channels for access into the stomach. The use of intraluminal techniques will undoubtedly be used to manage gastrointestinal and biliary disease without traditional open surgery.

IV. EXTRAPERITONEAL ACCESS

The extraperitoneal access to intraabdominal structures includes both the retroperitoneal and properitoneal approaches. Surgeons have long recognized that certain abdominal structures, (abdominal aorta, kidneys, and adrenal

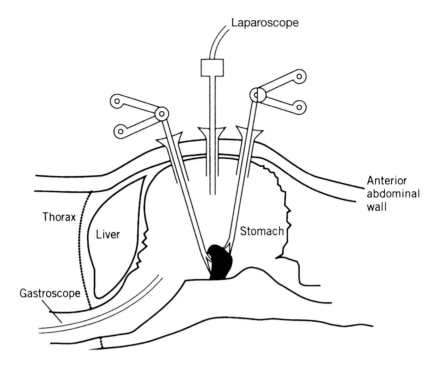

Figure 1.4. A diagram demonstrating intraluminal intragastric access.

glands) can be accessed extraperitoneally with better exposure than transperitoneally. Report of a prospective randomized trial comparing a transabdominal versus a retroperitoneal approach for abdominal aortic surgery has shown that the retroperitoneal approach resulted in shorter duration in both the intensive care unit and hospital with subsequent lower hospitalization costs.[8] Some vascular surgeons routinely perform aortic reconstructive surgery via the retroperitoneal approach in patients who have significant cardiopulmonary disease or who have had previous abdominal surgery (Table 1.1). But there are disadvantages that prohibit the wider acceptance of the retroperitoneal approach for aortic reconstructive surgery; for instance, access to the right renal and iliac arteries is difficult.

Adrenalectomy represents another use of the extraperitoneal approach to intraabdominal organs. Fahey and coworkers have successfully completed 47 out of 51 consecutive adrenalectomies via the extraperitoneal approach. The anterior approach was employed in three out of the four unsuccessful cases be-

TABLE 1.1

Advantages of the retroperitoneal approach

Allows use of regional anesthesia

Avoids creating intraabdominal adhesions

Decreases postoperative ileus

Lessens postoperative pain

Lessens postoperative pulmonary dysfunction

Minimizes third-space fluid loss

Permits development of clear dissection planes

cause of intraabdominal metastasis.[9] The retroperitoneal exposure for spine surgery results in less pain and the length of postoperative ileus.

Surgeons have used the properitoneal approach to perform laparoscopic herniorrhaphy.[10] The idea of properitoneal approach for hernia repair is not new: Cheatle in 1920 and Henry in 1936 used the properitoneal approach to repair inguinal and femoral hernias.[11,12] One major difference between Cheatle–Henry repair and modern laparoscopic repair is the introduction of synthetic material to repair the floor of the inguinal canal. Proponents of such an approach reason that this will avoid entering the abdomen during hernia repair, thereby reducing the risk of injuring intraabdominal organs and avoiding adhesions. The ideal candidates for laparoscopic herniorrhaphy are patients with bilateral inguinal defects, recurrent hernia, and simultaneous hernia repair in conjunction with other laparoscopic procedures.

New developments in balloon technology potentially will enable surgeons to perform retroperitoneal aortic surgery and spine surgery.[13,14] The balloon–dissection technique involves the initial placement of a small extraperitoneal incision for the insertion of the dissecting balloon. The balloon is then inflated and a laparoscope placed into the balloon dissector to create a working space in the retroperitoneum under direct laparoscopic guidance (Figure 1.5). Later, the dissecting balloon is removed and the retroperitoneal exposure is enlarged using either pneumoperitoneum or abdominal-wall retractor. Extraperitoneal procedures performed with open and laparoscopic techniques are listed in Table 1.2

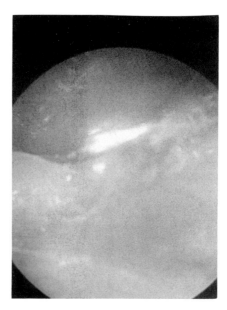

Figure 1.5. Retroperitoneal dissection using the dissecting balloon. The retroperitoneal space is carefully entered between the peritoneum and the retroperitoneum. The filmy area at the center of the picture is the retroperitoneal space being exposed by the dissecting balloon. (See insert for color representation.)

TABLE 1.2

Open and laparoscopic procedures previously performed via the properitoneal/retroperitoneal approach

Adrenalectomy

Aortic bypass

Bladder neck suspension

Inguinal and femoral hernia repair

Lumbar sympathectomy

Nephrectomy, ureterectomy

Retroperitoneal node-sampling

V. CONCLUSION

In the field of minimally invasive surgery, procedures that are routinely performed via a long incision may be replaced by access ports or miniincisions. The principles that have been developed and used in past years of open surgery to obtain access and exposure have not changed. In the following chapters, the various techniques of access into the abdomen, ranging from open to laparoscopic surgery will be discussed. An exciting phase of the evolution of laparoscopic surgery is the development of a gasless technique for the creation of the operating field, which has shown considerable promise and will be reviewed in detail in Chapters 7–10.

REFERENCES

1. Averbach M, Cohen RV, de Barros MV, et al.: "Laparoscopy assisted colonoscopic polypectomy." Surg Laparosc & Endosc 1995, 5:137–138.

2. Payne WG, Murphy CG, Grossbard LJ: "Combined laparoscopic and endoscopic approach to resection of gastric leiomyoma." J. Laparoendosc Surg 1995, 5:119–122.

3. Depaulo AL, Hashiba K, Bafutto M, et al.: "Laparoscopic antegrade sphincteromy." Surg Laparosc Endosc 1993, 3:157–160.

4. Gauderer MWL, Ponsky JL: "A simplified technique for constructing a tube feeding gastrostomy." Surg Gynecol Obstet 1981, 152:83–85.

5. Russell TR, Brotman M, Norris F: "Percutaneous gastrostomy—a new simplified and cost-effective technique." Am J Surg 1984, 132–137.

6. Ohashi S: "Laparoscopic intraluminal (intragastric) surgery for early gastric cancer. A new concept in laparoscopic surgery." Surg Endosc 1995, 9:169–171.

7. Filipi CJ, Perdikis G, Hinder RA, et al.: "An intraluminal surgical approach to the management of gastric bezoars." Surg Endosc 1995, 9:831–833.

8. Sicard GA, Reilly JM, Rubin BG, et al.: "Transabdominal versus retroperitoneal incision for abdominal aortic surgery: Report of a prospective randomized trial." J Vasc Surg 1995, 21:174–183.

9. Fahey TJ 3rd, Reeve TS, Delbridge L: "Adrenalectomy: expanded indications for the extraperitoneal approach." Aust N Z J Surg 1994, 64:494–497.

10. Phillips EH, Carroll BJ, Fallas MJ: "Laparoscopic preperitoneal inguinal hernia repair without peritoneal incision." Surg Endosc 1993, 7:159–162.

11. Cheatle, GL: "An operation for the radical cure of inguinal and femoral hernia." Br Med J 1920, 2:68–69.

12. Henry, AK: "Operation for femoral hernia by a midline extraperitoneal approach." Lancet 1936, 1:531–533.

13. Webb DR, Redgrave N, Chan Y, et al.: "Extraperitoneal laparoscopy: Early experience and evaluation." Aust N Z J Surg 1993, 63:554–557.

14. Himpens J, Van Alphen P, Cadiere GB, et al.: "Balloon dissection in extended retroperitoneoscopy." Surg Laparosc Endosc 1995, 5:193–196.

2

SURGICAL INCISIONS

Gerald W. Peskin, M.D.
Claude H. Organ, Jr., M.D.

I. INTRODUCTION

Until the era of minimal-access surgery, exposure at operation was obtained by a classic incision through the abdominal wall adequate to provide accessibility, extensibility, and security. The human eye was the camera, the overhead or headlamp light was the illuminating source, and the packs and retractors were the separators of contiguous structures from the site of manipulation. During the preoperative planning process, the surgeon took into account his or her own experience and training, the habitus of the patient, the probable accuracy of the diagnosis, and, perhaps, the potential cosmetic consequences. Rarely was there discussion of the cost of the procedure or the degree of pain experienced by the patient to justify one incision over another. Now the surgical journals are replete with articles suggesting virtual abolition of the wound, elimination of hospital stay (and cost), and, with the lessening of postoperative pain, an accelerated recovery and return to full activity. True, not all of the abdominal operative procedures are currently

Abdominal Access in Open and Laparoscopic Surgery
Edited by Edmund K. M. Tsoi and Claude H. Organ, Jr.
ISBN 0-471-13352-3 Copyright © 1996 by Wiley-Liss, Inc.

amenable to this minimalist approach, but perhaps this is only a function of time and surgical inventiveness.

To understand the placement of abdominal incisions, their current usefulness (in such situations as acute abdominal problems, peritonitis, previously explored abdomens, pregnancy, and lesions inaccessible to laparoscopic removal), amelioration of the temporary disability the incisions produce, as well as their complications, it is important to review the dynamics of the anterior abdominal wall.

II. DYNAMICS OF THE ANTERIOR ABDOMINAL WALL

The abdominal wall is largely muscular and extends between the bony pelvis and thorax. This wall moves the trunk and provides a girdle-like compression of the abdominal contents. Three pairs of muscles are broad and flat (internal/external obliques and transversus) and form the major part of the anterolateral abdominal wall, while the strap-like rectus abdominis, situated on either side of the midline, and the pyramidalis, embedded in the rectus sheath just above the pubis, provide central strength and the ability to flex the trunk on the pelvis and vice versa. The segmental nervous innervation enters laterally from lower thoracic segments (to the first lumbar nerve), slanting forward obliquely toward the midline. The main branches of these nerves run between the internal oblique and transversus muscles. Lateral cutaneous branches from corresponding posterior and subcostal vessels accompany the nerves with perforating anterior cutaneous vessels derived from the longitudinally running channel—superior and inferior epigastrics. The midline of the abdominal wall is secured by the linea alba, a multilaminated fascial structure, which binds the rectus sheaths together and is widest at the umbilicus, diminishing in width as it approaches the xiphoid. It is free of gross nervous or vascular branches, but is under the greatest stress from the competing pull of the flat muscles of each side.

III. CHOICE OF ABDOMINAL INCISIONS

Before an incision is made, it must be planned. General considerations include the organs and disease process to be evaluated, the habitus of the patient, the necessity for speed, the presence of previous abdominal incisions, the potential extent of the operation anticipated, and, of course, the surgeon's individual preference. Following this accounting, there are a number of factors to keep in mind, as outlined by Skandalakis:[3]

1. The incision should be adequate, long enough for a good exposure and for room to work, and short enough to avoid unnecessary complications.

2. Skin incisions should follow Langer's lines where possible.

3. Avoid incisions parallel to existing scars (excise the scar and proceed).

4. Muscles should be split in the direction of their fibers rather than transected (an exception is the rectus muscle which, because of its segmental nerve supply, can be transected).

5. Where possible, the openings formed through the different layers of the abdominal wall should not be superimposed.

6. Avoid cutting nerves wherever possible.

7. Muscles and abdominal organs should be retracted toward, not away from, their neurovascular supply.

8. Drains should be inserted through separate small incisions, not in the primary wound.

9. Cosmetic considerations must be afforded close attention, but the principles of accessibility, extensibility, and security must prevail.

The tensile strength of the anterior abdominal wall rests in its fascial–aponeurotic layers. Tensionometer readings in experimental animals before and after removal of the rectus abdominis reveal no significant difference. When the flat muscles of the abdomen contract, the wound edges of a transverse incision are approximated by the vector forces of these muscles. In vertical incisions, these same actions coupled with contraction of the rectus muscles, tend to separate these wound margins.

Most commonly, three types of incisions are used to explore the abdominal cavity:[1]

Vertical. These may be midline (median) or paramedian and supra- or infraumbilical, lending themselves well to extension up or down. Vertical

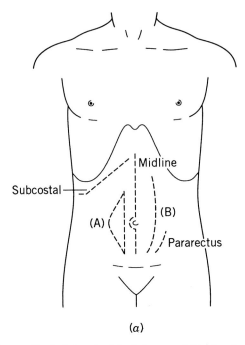

Figure 2.1*a*. Major vertical abdominal incisions and Kocher (subcostal) incision. (A) Paramedian incision with rectus muscle retraction. (B) Paramedian incision with rectus muscle split.

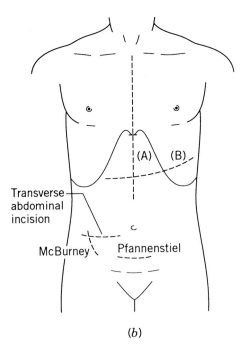

Figure 2.1*b*. Major transverse abdominal and thoraco–abdominal incisions. (A) With sternal split, (B) with rib division.

16

incisions, except for the midline, place more anterior wall nerves and arteries at risk than do transverse incisions.

Transverse and Oblique. These are exemplified by the McBurney incision for appendectomy, the Kocher subcostal incision for cholecystectomy, and the Pfannenstiel incision commonly employed in gynecologic operations.

Thoracoabdominal. These are employed for extensive exposure of the liver and esophagogastric juncture (Figure 2.1*b*).

Though oblique and transverse incisions are more tedious to perform, surgeons have preferentially advocated their use on the grounds that they are stronger and less liable to herniate or disrupt. The same has been said for paramedian incisions. However, after many controlled trials and retrospective reviews, it is apparent that, when similar techniques of closure and similar suture material are used, no significant difference is noted in the major sequelae (dehiscence and herniation) caused by the various types of incisions. Similarly, when the same suture material was used and only the technique (interrupted versus continuous) was varied, no significant variation in sequelae resulted, regardless of the types of incisions compared. Only the use of absorbable as opposed to nonabsorbable sutures for the closure appeared to result in a greater tendency to herniation. While a transverse abdominal incision closed in interrupted fashion with nonabsorbable sutures should theoretically be the most secure combination, the ultimate decision by the operating surgeon is based more on the tenets noted in the introductory part of this section.

IV. INDIVIDUAL INCISIONS

Midline

Almost all operations in the abdomen or retroperitoneum can be performed through this incision, which can be made and closed quickly, is almost bloodless, and divides no muscle fibers. Extension from the xiphoid to the pubis is possible (or the xiphoid may be removed) and extension into the mediastinum and/or thorax can be easily achieved. In some individuals a well-vascularized fatty layer may accompany the peritoneum in the upper midline. This layer can be avoided by reflecting the rectus fascia to either side and entering the peritoneum somewhat left lateral of center where minimal or no fat has infiltrated. The falciform ligament (ligamentum teres) is easily avoided but can be ligated and divided if encountered. Splenectomy, hiatus hernia repair, vagotomy, gastric resection, antireflux procedures, pancreatectomy, and biliary and liver operations can all be done through the upper portion of a midline incision, whereas abdominal aortic reconstruction and colonic and gynecologic procedures are easily performed through the lower reaches of the midline approach. (Watch out for bladder!)

Paramedian

Theoretically, this incision has several advantages over the midline approach, among which are that closure may be more secure because the rectus muscle acts as a buttress between the reapproximated anterior and posterior fascial planes, and access to lateral structures on the right or left may be easier. In fact, neither of these advantages is of great import. The skin incision is placed 2–5 cm lateral to the midline and once the anterior rectus sheath is incised, its medial portion is dissected free of rectus muscle. Thereupon, the rectus muscle mass is retracted laterally and the posterior sheath and peritoneum are incised vertically in the same anteroposterior plane as the anterior fascial incision. When utilized in the lower abdomen, the deep inferior epigastric vessels are encountered and need to be ligated and divided if they interfere with the posterior incision. Some surgeons prefer to split the rectus muscle, rather than dissect it free and displace it laterally, which causes atrophy of the muscle body medial to the incision. Others like to curve the incision toward the xiphoid in its upper reaches rather than straight to the costal margin (Mayo–Robson extension). Closure may be in layers or with a full-thickness technique. The span of access to intraabdominal viscera is comparable to that achieved by the midline incision.

Kocher Subcostal

This subcostal incision offers excellent exposure for the biliary passages and gallbladder, and when utilized on the left side affords access to the spleen. It is of particular value in obese and unduly muscular patients. Starting in the midline about 2 fingerbreadths (2.5–5 cm) below the xiphoid, the incision parallels the costal margin, remaining at least 2.5 cm below it. The length, usually about 12–15 cm, is determined by the body habitus of the patient. The anterior rectus sheath is incised in the same direction as the skin incision and the rectus muscle is divided. The posterior sheath and transversus abdominis muscle are split with attention to the superior epigastric vessels, which enter the sheath at the level of the ninth costal cartilage. The lateral musculature is cut in an outward direction, sparing both the ninth dorsal nerve to prevent weakness of the abdominal wall and the tenth dorsal nerve to avoid umbilical paresthesia. The incision is then deepened to open the peritoneum. It may be carried further across the midline into an inverted V configuration, adding to the exposure for upper abdominal organs. One side of the incision may be longer than the other, depending on the need for exposure. The rectus muscle can be cut transversely without creating serious abdominal-wall weakness, provided its anterior and posterior sheaths are appropriately reapproximated during closure. Healing of the rectus muscle wound results simply in the formation of an additional tendinous inscription.

Transverse Muscle-Dividing

This incision can be used at almost any level of the abdominal wall to expose intraabdominal structures by dividing all the tissues underlying the skin incision. The technique is similar to that described for the Kocher incision. It is useful in newborns and infants and in adults who are short and obese because it creates more abdominal exposure per unit length than do vertical incisions.

McBurney (Muscle-Splitting)

Devised in the late nineteenth century, this incision is frequently employed in operations for suspected acute appendicitis. It offers very good access and can be readily extended and quickly closed with a nice cosmetic result. Classically, the skin incision is made at the junction of the middle and outer thirds of a line running from the umbilicus to the anterior superior iliac spine. Originally, the incision was placed obliquely from above laterally to below medially. However many surgeons now use a transverse incision in a skin crease for improved cosmetic results (Rockey–Davis incision for appendectomy). The external oblique aponeurosis is then split in the direction of its fibers, the lateral border of the rectus muscle located, and the internal oblique and transversus muscle fibers are separately bluntly from the rectus border laterally toward the iliac crest with minimal damage. A fold of peritoneum is grasped, elevated, and opened. Further access can be easily obtained by dividing the anterior rectus sheath medially in line with the internal oblique incision, after which the rectus muscle may be either retracted medially or divided. Lateral extension can be achieved by dividing and splitting the oblique muscles along the lines of their fibers in the lateral direction. In addition to the right-sided incision, a similar approach in the left lower abdomen can be useful in dealing with lesions of the sigmoid colon. Closure is simple: the muscle bellies reapproximate themselves after the peritoneum and transversus muscle edges are brought together; the major layer approximation is the external oblique. There is no need to close the flat muscles in this incision because reapproximation sutures may cause liqueficative necrosis of the ilio–inguinal and iliohypogastric nerves and affect the shutter mechanism of the internal inguinal ring.

Pfannenstiel

Popular with gynecologists and urologists, this incision affords access to the pelvic organs and retropubic space. The skin is incised for about 5 inches in a fold approximately 2 inches above the symphysis pubis (within the hair line), and the incision then deepened to expose both rectus sheaths. Following division of both sheaths along the entire length of the incision, the rectus sheaths are freed from the underlying rectus muscles, umbilicus to pubis. The rectus muscles are then separated in the midline and retracted laterally and the peritoneum is opened vertically in the midline with care to avoid bladder injury. An excellent cosmetic result is ensured, but exposure is limited and this approach should not be used when a procedure outside the pelvis might be necessary.

Thoracoabdominal

These incisions convert the pleural and peritoneal cavities into a common cavity, affording excellent exposure for major right-sided hepatic operations or for the lower left-sided esophageal and stomach procedures. After appropriate positioning of the abdomen and thorax, the peritoneal cavity is opened through a vertical incision in the upper abdomen and preliminary exploration performed. The incision may then be extended along the line of the eighth interspace (just caudad to inferior pole of the scapula). If an oblique upper-abdominal incision is used, it may be continued directly into the thoracic portion of the incision. With the abdomen opened, the chest incision is deepened through the latissimus dorsi, serratus anterior, external oblique, and intercostal muscles to enter the pleural cavity. The incision is continued across the costal margin (a short segment may be resected). The diaphragm is divided radially after ligation of inferior phrenic vessel branches. Closure techniques vary, but pleural cavity drainage through a separate stab incision and secure reapproximation of the costal margin are important to all methods.

With the advent of the laparoscopic approach have come advances in instrumentation and much thought about the immediate consequences of standard incisions of the abdominal wall. One can utilize the videoscope to aid in dissection of difficult areas through smaller incisions and devise small incisions such as those in the "minimal-stress triangle," the lateral sides of which are formed by the medial margins of the sixth through eighth costochondral cartilages within the subxiphoid areas and the base of which is formed by a plane joining the eighth costal cartilages. In this triangle, the anterior abdominal-wall movements are limited and pain minimized so that cholecystectomy

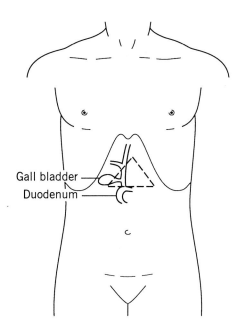

Figure 2.2. Triangle of minimal stress (see ref. 4).

can be carried out through a 3-cm incision, videoscopically aided and using conventional instrumentation. In this fashion, cholecystectomy becomes an outpatient procedure, with no more need for postoperative analgesia than that required for standard laparoscopic cholecystectomy. No doubt other unique approaches to intraabdominal viscera will be devised, limited only by surgeons' ingenuity (Figure 2.2).[4]

V. COMPLICATIONS OF ABDOMINAL INCISIONS

The most common and troublesome problems associated with abdominal incisions include poor exposure, accidental injury of viscera, infection, dehiscence, evisceration, incisional hernia, pain, and complaints of unsightliness, numbness, and being able to feel the sutures.[2]

The primary goal of every abdominal incision is to provide exposure sufficient for the safe and easy conduct of the contemplated procedure; this principle must never be compromised. Severe complications may follow a misplaced or inadequate wound, such as those that can be noted with repair of ureteral injuries through too high an opening; truncal vagotomy and esophageal operations through incisions that are too low; and missed pathology through too small a wound. In general, emergency celiotomy for trauma should be performed through a midline incision to cope with the unpredictable; the liver, biliary tract, pancreas, and spleen are most easily exposed through subcostal incisions; stomach, proximal duodenum, and intraabdominal esophagus visualization calls for a high (to the top of the xiphoid) midline approach by most surgeons; and procedures deep in the pelvis require a lower midline approach for safety. If the patient is thin and has a narrow subcostal angle, a transverse incision has no advantage, whereas if the patient is obese with a wide subcostal angle, an oblique or transverse incision provides excellent upper-abdominal access. Overall, no matter what the direction of an incision, its length must be ample.

Accidental injury to viscera may occur in several ways. The three most common opportunities for injury to take place are when the peritoneum is opened (especially when adhesions are present), when retractors are positioned, and when suture penetration occurs during closure of the peritoneum and fascia. To prevent these injuries from occurring, the patient must be completely relaxed so that he will not struggle and inadvertently move intraabdominal viscera into the wound. In addition, careful, sharp dissection in a bloodless field is needed to reveal appropriate planes to separate viscera, retractor blades must be protected with moist pads and kept at the correct tension by an alert assistant or mechanical device, and the peritoneum should be exposed and elevated with forceps prior to the incision.

Most abdominal-incision infections are superficial, confined to the subcutaneous fat. However, following an operation involving peritonitis or fecal spill, a local infection may contaminate fascia and muscle or a small number of wounds may be invaded by synergistic, clostridial, or other combined organisms that destroy healthy tissue. Vulnerability to these infections is enhanced by the presence of hematomas, seromas, mass ligatures, devitalized tissue, strangulating sutures, dead space, and obesity. Cardinal symptoms of infection are pain, tenderness, swelling, redness, and discharge with signs of temperature elevation and leucocytosis. Infection can usually be managed by wound care with debridement, irrigation, and packing. Antibiotics are reserved for evidence of invasive manifestations or for a prosthesis requiring protection. Where necrotizing myositis or fasciitis is suspected or apparent, radical debridement of destroyed tissue along with intravenous antibiotics are mandatory until normal margins are noted. Overall, one should not tolerate an infection rate of over 2% with abdominal incisions.

Dehiscence of an abdominal wound may occur with or without evisceration. In general, when the dehiscence is small and infection is present, evisceration may not be an issue due to the adherence of inflamed viscera to each other and to the parietal peritoneum. Dehiscence and infection are best dealt with by local cleansing and adherent dressing until covered with healthy granulation. If the defect in the fascia is large enough to threaten evisceration, repair is necessary. Dehiscence without infection occurs on the fifth to tenth day after the operation, just after skin sutures have been removed. This type of dehiscence is signaled by the release of serosanguineous fluid from the wound and the appearance of the small bowel and omentum on the abdominal wall. Occurring in about 1% of laparotomy incisions (although an incidence of up to 10% has been reported), this complication carries a significant mortality (15%), and requires immediate repair with nonabsorbable sutures. Predisposing factors for this infection include malnutrition, uremia, anemia, shock, liver failure, obesity, advanced age, distention (ileus), straining due to coughing and vomiting, wound tension, convulsions, and technical problems during closure. Although most eviscerations occur through midline incisions, there is no evidence to prove that midline incisions in adults are more liable to eviscerate than other incisions. (This is explained by the frequent need for midline incisions in severely injured, septic, starved, and cancer-ridden patients.) Nor is there evidence to show that dehiscence is more frequent in continuous as opposed to interrupted suturing techniques. Only the use of nonabsorbable instead of absorbable sutures (catgut) results in fewer dehiscences. No technique gives perfect protection, although attention to details, such as including a large mass of tissue in each stitch and tying without strangulation, is paramount. Late repair of hernias is necessary where initial fascial closure was not attempted or was unsuccessful.

Pain is an inevitable consequence of abdominal incisions. The response to surgical trauma of the abdominal wall involves nociceptive input arising from the skin and somatic structures. Skin damage produces a sharp, well-localized sensation. Somatic damage manifests itself in pain around the incision or in a referred area of pain that is more diffuse and aching. The tissue injury sets up responses at the spinal-cord level corresponding to the site of injury. These responses include skeletal muscle spasm, vasospasm, ischemia, and release of algesic substances. Stimulation of the brain stem and diencephalon, mostly through lateral ascending spinal tracts, activates autonomic responses such as ventilation, circulation, sympathetic output, and hypothalamic endocrine release. Cortical projections perceive pain. This perception initiates voluntary skeletal muscle activity and contributes to emotional responses. Postoperative pain is influenced by preoperative preparation; emotional, psychological and motivational factors; the site and nature of the operation; and the type and location of the incision. In general, two days of constant pain and about a week of pain on motion are the usual effects of every laparotomy incision. Pain is greatest in vertical abdominal incisions because they are subject to traction by the flat muscles from both sides of the abdominal wall. Pain is less in transverse and oblique incisions, especially muscle-splitting. Lower abdominal wounds are not influenced by respiratory excursions as much as are upper abdominal incisions and thus are less painful.

As a means of alleviating postoperative distress, one may employ an intramuscular, intravenous, oral, or spinal drug or combinations of these agents, making sure to maintain a therapeutic level and to sustain analgesia between doses and changing the drug if relief is not satisfactory. Since the risk of producing iatrogenic addiction is low in postsurgical patients, adequate dosage to control pain should be paramount in the surgeon's orders. Patient-controlled analgesia (PCA) with a loading dose, incremental subsequent doses to maintain therapeutic levels, a lockout interval between doses, and a set maximum for the time period between doses have greatly aided postoperative drug utilization. Spinal and/or epidural opiate administration, although more cumbersome and reserved for in-patients, has proven very effective for pain relief. Finally, long-acting local anesthetics that provide several hours of relief and reduce the need for systemic therapy can be administered by the surgeon at the conclusion of the procedure.

Coupled with all of these methods of pain relief is the knowledge that attention to patient care through instruction and encouragement can reduce the need for narcotics, make the patient more comfortable physically and emotionally, and thus shorten hospital stay. There is no question that larger incisions produce more pain than smaller ones, but with proper pain management, the difference may not be as great as is often thought.

No matter how corrective or even life-sparing your operation, some patients will complain to you about the color or size of their scars. Some truly have keloid formation; some merely have hypertrophy requiring time for resolution. Some patients are uncomfortable about the numbness that may be present distal to nerve transection. Some may notice pain associated with suture knots, especially thin patients when slippable suture material is used. Some may think they have abnormal bulging in the wound area. And the complaints go on! It is important to assure yourself and the patient, through the use of appropriate examination and testing, that the problem is not one of recurrent or new visceral disorders, that the wound is secure, and that remedies are not to be found in surgical manipulation.

VI. CONCLUSIONS

Despite the advances in laparoscopic techniques, there will always be a need for open surgical approaches to the abdomen. It thus behooves the general surgeon to understand the pros and cons of the various incisions noted above. Perhaps in this new era of competition between laparoscopy and open surgery, we will become more aware of problems associated with open abdominal operations, such as pain, cosmesis, infection and failure of proper healing, and through this awareness reduce the incidence of these sequelae to the benefit of our patients.

REFERENCES

1. Ellis H: "Abdominal wall: Incisions and closures." In Schwartz SI, Ellis H, (eds.), Maingot's Abdominal Operations. 9th ed. Norwalk, CT: Appleton and Lange, 1989, 179–193.

2. McGuire HH Jr.: "Complications of abdominal wall surgery." In Greenfield LJ, (ed.), Complications in Surgery and Trauma. 2d ed. Philadelphia, PA: Lippincott, 1990, 490–498.

3. Skandalakis JE, Gray SW, Rowe JS Jr.: "Incisions of the anterior abdominal wall." In Anatomical Complications in General Surgery. New York, NY: McGraw-Hill, 1983, 292–301.

4. Tyagi NS, Meredith MC, Lumb JC, et al.: "A new minimally invasive technique for cholecystectomy: Subxiphoid 'minimal stress triangle' microceliotomy." Ann Surg 1994, 220:617–525.

3

TECHNIQUES OF CO$_2$ PNEUMOPERITONEUM

Vernon J. Henderson, M.D.

I. TECHNIQUES OF CO$_2$ PNEUMOPERITONEUM

The traditional approach to establishing pneumoperitoneum for laparoscopy was introduced by Semm in 1964.[1] This technique involves the establishment of a pneumoperitoneum in the periumbilical region as a convenient site where the abdominal wall is relatively thin and the area is free of significant blood vessels. Several preparatory measures are undertaken prior to establishing a pneumoperitoneum. To maximize the safety of this approach, the bladder is decompressed with a catheter to prevent inadvertent injury to the distended bladder. Intermittent compression stockings should be placed on the patient prior to induction of anesthesia and activated as soon as the patient is paralyzed, since they have been shown to overcome or diminish the hemodynamic consequences of pneumoperitoneum.[2,3] Distention of the abdomen with carbon dioxide has been shown to decrease venous return to the heart by as much as 50% and is associated with distention of the femoral veins, which reflects increased lower extremity venous pressures.[4] Intermittent compression stock-

Abdominal Access in Open and Laparoscopic Surgery
Edited by Edmund K. M. Tsoi and Claude H. Organ, Jr.
ISBN 0-471-13352-3 Copyright © 1996 by Wiley-Liss, Inc.

ings have been shown to lessen the hemodynamic effects of pneumoperitoneum.[2,3]

A semicircular incision is made in the periumbilical area beginning either above or below the umbilicus. This incision is deepened to the level of the fascia with blunt dissection using a small clamp. Pneumoperitoneum can be established by a closed method using a needle to access the peritoneal cavity, or by an open method that allows direct visualization and placement of a cannula into the peritoneal cavity.

The closed technique for establishing pneumoperitoneum involves the introduction of air into the peritoneal cavity through a needle to initially distend the abdomen after which a trocar can be safely inserted through the distended abdominal wall.[5] To accomplish this technique, vertical traction is applied to the anterior abdominal wall by placing upward traction on towel clips applied to the corners of the periumbilical incision. This maneuver adds a margin of safety to the procedure by causing a release of the intestine from the anterior abdominal wall upon introducing air through the Veress needle. The needle is introduced through the intact fascia. With good vertical traction and modern retractable needle tips a palpable "pop" can be felt upon entry of the needle into the free peritoneal space. Verification of intraperitoneal needle placement is obtained by connecting a syringe to the needle and aspirating to establish whether there is return of bile or intestinal contents. If this procedure produces no intestinal contents, a small amount of water is injected through the needle, and the syringe is removed from the needle. Upon removing the syringe, the fluid meniscus should rapidly drop into the peritoneal cavity, indicating the free flow of fluid into the peritoneal space. At this point, the needle can be connected to the insufflation source and the flow of carbon dioxide through the needle and into the peritoneal space can begin.

The initial flow of CO$_2$ should be at a low rate in case the needle was inadvertently placed into the lumen of the bowel or outside the peritoneal cavity. This is indicated by a rapid rise in the pressure reading at the insufflator. Appropriate placement in the free peritoneal cavity is indicated by gradual distention of the abdomen at low intraabdominal pressures initially; pressures rise as abdominal distention occurs. Once a satisfactory level of abdominal distention has been obtained (intraabdominal pressures of approximately 15 mm Hg), the Veress needle can be removed. At this point, an appropriately sized trocar can be introduced through the periumbilical incision. A trocar large enough to accommodate the laparoscope is placed blindly through the abdominal wall, the laparoscope is then introduced through this trocar so that all remaining trocars can be placed under direct vision.

The closed technique for creation of a CO$_2$ pneumoperitoneum has several advantages. The technique is fast, relatively safe, and because the trocar is introduced through the anterior abdominal wall, a tight seal around the trocar can be obtained. The Veress needle is much less traumatic to the anterior abdominal wall and is also less traumatic to bowel or other intraabdominal structures in the event of an inadvertent injury to these areas. The closed technique using the Veress needle is still fraught with potential hazards, and some authors caution against its use in laparoscopic abdominal operations.[6] While it is less traumatic than placing the trocar blindly into an undistended abdomen, the reduced dangers are a matter of degree rather than absolute.[7] The potential complications associated with the Veress needle are similar to those of blind trocar placement.[7] Injuries to intraabdominal viscera, including the bowel and bladder, have been reported with the use of the Veress needle, as well as injuries to major vascular structures.

The open technique for establishing pneumoperitoneum was introduced by Hasson to address the dangers related to the closed technique. The open technique allows placement of a modified trocar directly into the peritoneal cavity through a small incision, using the same initial approach as the closed technique. The abdominal wall fascia is identified and grasped between clamps or forceps, and the fascia and peritoneum are incised under direct vision. When the trocar is placed in the abdominal cavity, the surgeon inserts his or her finger to establish that the anterior abdominal wall is free of adhesions. A pursestring suture of a heavy material is then placed in the fascia and peritoneum, and the cannula is introduced into the abdominal cavity through the pursestring. The pursestring suture is tied securely around the cannula to obtain an airtight closure. Carbon dioxide is then introduced through the cannula to a point where adequate abdominal distention has been obtained at an intraabdominal pressure of approximately 15 mm Hg.

The advantage of the open technique is the safety associated with placement of the trocar under direct vision.[6] It is more difficult to maintain an airtight seal with the open technique, since a larger opening in the fascia and peritoneum is required; however, with proper placement of a heavy pursestring suture that can be tightened successfully about the trocar, an airtight seal can be obtained with relative ease.

Once the periumbilical trocar has been placed, by open or closed technique, the laparoscope can be introduced and the other trocars can be placed at other sites under direct vision. Additional trocars are placed directly through small skin incisions. The laparoscope is used to directly observe each trocar entry into the distended abdominal cavity. Trocar placement for specific operative procedures will be discussed in detail.

The pneumoperitoneum is maintained throughout the operative procedure by the CO$_2$ insufflator, which maintains intraabdominal pressure at a preset level. All sites of penetration of the anterior abdominal wall are sealed tightly to prevent leaks of gas from the abdomen, but some loss of intraabdominal gas is inevitable. As CO$_2$ escapes from the abdominal cavity or is absorbed into the circulation, it is replaced by the insufflator to maintain intraabdominal pressure. Intraabdominal pressure is typically maintained at approximately 15 mm Hg for most laparoscopic procedures. This pressure represents a compromise between the poor exposure of intraabdominal structures afforded by lower intraabdominal pressures and the adverse hemodynamic consequences of higher pressures.[4,8-10] Furthermore, venous return is compromised by high intraabdominal pressure. At operating pressures of 15 mm Hg, venous return through the inferior vena cava is reduced by approximately 50%. Additionally, CO$_2$ absorption is significantly increased requiring higher minute ventilation to maintain normal arterial CO$_2$ levels.[4,11]

At the end of the operative procedure the pneumoperitoneum is released and the CO$_2$ is allowed to escape from the abdominal cavity. An active attempt is made to remove all gas from the abdominal cavity to prevent continued CO$_2$ absorption through the peritoneal cavity. The patient may also develop shoulder pain resulting from CO$_2$ accumulation under the leaves of the diaphragm.[12]

Gases other than carbon dioxide have been used in the past to establish pneumoperitoneum. Room air, oxygen, helium, and nitrous oxide have all been used for pneumoperitoneum, but these gases has been abandoned because of their potential risk of combustion or other safety issues.[13,14] Air and pure oxygen carry an obvious combustion risk due to the presence of oxygen, a highly combustible gas. Nitrous oxide, by comparison, carries little inherent risk of combustion, but two case reports exist in the literature of explosions occurring under unusual circumstances in the presence of nitrous oxide. In both cases it is presumed that either methane or hydrogen produced by colonic bacteria were responsible for the explosions.[13] These gases became combustible when they attain certain concentrations in the abdominal cavity in the presence of nitrous oxide. Methane and hydrogen are byproducts of bacterial metabolism in the colon and, theoretically, nitrous oxide could never be used in laparoscopic colon procedures due to the potential of large amounts of methane or hydrogen being released into the peritoneal cavity when the colon is opened.

A recent study casts some doubt on the combustion risk associated with methane or hydrogen accumulation during laparoscopic cholecystectomy performed with carbon dioxide pneumoperitoneum.[13] Further investigation of this phenomenon is necessary before nitrous oxide can be advocated safely for routine use during laparoscopic surgery. At this time carbon dioxide fits the bill as the most practical agent for establishing pneumoperitoneum. It is inexpensive, readily absorbed, rapidly eliminated, and suppresses combustion. The potential severe cardiovascular side effects associated with carbon dioxide pneumoperitoneum has increased interest in seeking other methods for creating pneumoperitoneum.[15] Helium is one gas that may offer significant advantages over carbon dioxide.[11]

II. ACCESS FOR SPECIFIC OPERATIONS

Laparoscopic Cholecystectomy

Laparoscopic cholecystectomy is the most common laparoscopic operation performed by general surgeons.[16,17] Since its introduction in 1988, laparoscopic cholecystectomy has become the procedure of choice for managing cholelithiasis.[18] The patient is placed supine on the operating table and video monitors, light sources, and the insufflator are positioned for optimal viewing by the surgeons. The surgeon performs this operation typically from the left side of the patient. The first assistant typically stands to the patient's right.[19]

Access for this procedure typically begins by establishing pneumoperitoneum using carbon dioxide (Figure 3.1). Pneumoperitoneum can be established by either the open or closed technique. An intraabdominal pressure of approximately 15 mm Hg is obtained prior to placement of trocars, and this pressure is maintained throughout the procedure.

The initial periumbilical port is placed as previously described. Additional ports are placed in the right upper quadrant in the midclavicular line, the right lower quadrant in the anterior axillary line, and in the epigastrium to

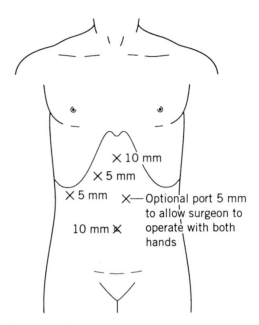

Figure 3.1. Laparoscopic cholecystectomy.

allow mobilization and dissection of the gallbladder. The epigastric port is generally placed under direct vision following placement of the umbilical port and laparoscope. A 10-mm port is placed in the epigastrium. The port may be directed through the avascular portion of the falciform ligament or it may bypass the falciform ligament altogether. The epigastric port is used by the surgeon as a primary port for dissection of the porta hepatis. The gallbladder can be grasped or simply exposed to allow a grasping instrument to be placed from another site.

Additional 5-mm ports are then placed in the right upper quadrant in the mid-clavicular line and in the right lower quadrant in the mid-axillary line to grasp and manipulate the gallbladder. A fourth 5-mm port can be placed in the left mid abdomen to allow the surgeon to operate with both hands. Exposure of the gallbladder fossa is facilitated by placing the operating table in reverse Trendelenburg position to allow gravity to assist in moving the colon and small bowel out of the operative field.

At the end of the procedure the trocars can be removed and the pneumoperitoneum can be released actively by aspiration through an abdominal suction apparatus and by application of external pressure to the abdominal wall to force gas from the peritoneal cavity through the trocar sites. The trocar sites can then be closed in a standard fashion by reapproximating the fascia with a suitable suture; the skin can be closed with sutures, staples, or Steri-strips™.

Nissen Fundoplication

Extension of laparoscopic techniques to antireflux operations has developed rapidly over the past four to five years.[20] Many centers have gained significant clinical experience with laparoscopic antireflux operations, and reports are beginning to appear in the literature that compare laparoscopic operations to open antireflux operations in randomized prospective trials.[21–24] Laparoscopic antireflux surgery is attractive from a theoretical perspective and its application offers patients the proven superior efficacy of operative therapy for gastroesophageal reflux while sparing patients the operative morbidity of conventional open fundoplication. As more reports of the successful application of laparoscopic fundoplication appear in the literature, it is becoming more obvious that these theoretical advantages are clinically obtainable.

A recent comparative report concludes that symptomatic outcome is similar for laparoscopic fundoplication and open fundoplication. Laparoscopic fundoplication may provide greater augmentation of lower esophageal sphincter pressure in addition to the commonly described advantages of less postoperative pain and shorter hospital stays.[24]

Several different laparoscopic approaches to antireflux operations that have been described differ in positioning of the patient and the operating surgeon and in placement of the operative ports.[21,23–25] Technical variations have also been reported that allow easier access and dissection of the gastroesophageal junction and control of the short gastric vessels. Laparoscopic fundoplication is generally performed from an anterior abdominal approach with the patient supine; the surgeon stands either to the patient's left or between the patient's legs, and operative trocars are variously placed in the upper abdominal quadrants.

Cuschieri and associates[23] perform fundoplication with the patient in the supine position and the surgeon standing to the patient's left side. Pneumoperitoneum is established through an open or closed technique and the laparoscope is placed through an 11-mm cannula placed 3 cm above and to the left of the umbilicus. Other trocars are placed below and to the right of the xiphoid process, 4 cm to the right and above the umbilicus, midway between the xiphoid and the umbilicus, and at the lower edge of the left subcostal region (Figure 3.2).

Fontaumard et al.[26] have recently reported successful Nissen–Rossetti fundoplication in 148 patients with symptomatic gastroesophageal reflux without a conversion or postoperative death. The patient is operated on in the lithotomy position and pneumoperitoneum is established by the closed technique in the midclavicular line below the left costal margin. Four 10-mm ports are placed as follows: one each in the midclavicular line in the left subcostal area, in the subxiphoid region, in the supraumbilical area, and in the left mid-abdominal area. A 5-mm trocar is placed in the right subcostal region to assist in exposing the gastroesophageal junction (Figure 3.3).

Snow and associates[27] perform a "physiologic reconstruction" of the gastroesophageal anatomy with the patient in the supine position and the surgeon standing to the patient's left. The laparoscope is inserted through a 10-mm port placed 1–2 inches above the umbilicus. Ten-millimeter ports are placed in the right and left subcostal areas. Two 5-mm working ports are placed in the

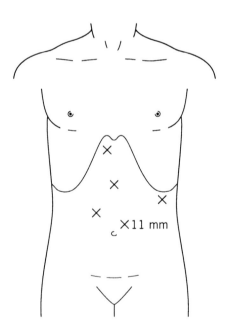

Figure 3.2. Nissen fundoplication.[23]

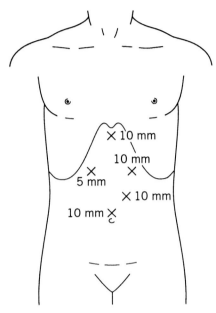

Figure 3.3. Nissen-Rosetti fundoplication.[26]

right and left upper abdominal quadrants to facilitate dissection of the gastroe-sophageal junction (Figure 3.4).

Laparoscopic procedures to repair paraesophageal hernias and to relieve obstruction due to esophageal achalasia have been described. These proce-dures employ sight variations on the techniques established for performing fundoplication to expose the gastroesophageal junction and paraesophageal areas.[28–30]

Large Bowel Resection

Laparoscopic colectomy was first reported in 1990 as a natural extension of the experience gained with laparoscopic cholecystectomy to other abdominal pro-cedures.[31] Laparoscopic colon resections are generally considered "laparoscop-ic-assisted" since the abdominal wall must be opened, if only through a small incision, to remove the specimen and to assist in the colon anastomosis. Lap-aroscopic-assisted procedures may employ laparoscopy to simply mobilize the lateral peritoneal attachments of the colon[32] or the full operation from mobi-

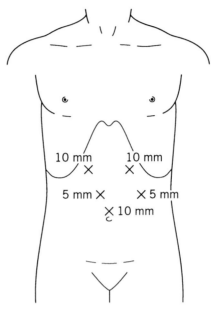

Figure 3.4. **Physiologic reconstruction of GE junction.**[27]

lization of the colon to intracorporeal anastomosis of the colon may be performed with laparoscopic technique.[32–34] A larger incision is eventually made in the abdominal wall for removal of the colon specimen and/or anastomosis of the remaining colon. Laparoscopic techniques differ depending on the extent and location of the segment of colon to be removed; these techniques have been reported to facilitate resection of all portions of the accessible colon and rectum.[32–39]

   Wexner and colleagues reported one of the first prospective comparisons of laparoscopic total abdominal colectomy and standard open total colectomy for patients with the following diagnoses: mucosal ulcerative colitis, familial polyposis coli, or colonic inertia.[38] The study group underwent laparoscopic colon mobilization. The colon was removed and the extracorporeal anastomosis was performed through a small lower midline or modified Pfannenstiel incision. The laparoscopic portion of the procedure was performed using pneumoperitoneum established through a standard umbilical approach with trocars placed in the upper and lower abdominal regions as necessary to complete mobilization of the colon.

   Recent reports describe the use of colonoscopy to assist in laparoscopic colon mobilization to improve exposure and facilitate dissection of the splenic and hepatic flexures of the colon.[35] Pneumoperitoneum is utilized for the laparoscopic portion of the colon resection.

A multicenter prospective, nonrandomized trial of laparoscopic versus open colon resection for adenocarcinoma involving 194 patients was recently reported. Results suggest that, when compared to open colon resection, laparoscopic colon resection for cancer allows a comparable resection with adequate margins and equivalent recovery of mesenteric lymph nodes. Early follow-up suggests comparable survival and disease-free intervals.[34]

Laparoscopic colon resection for malignant conditions has been less readily accepted than laparoscopic colon removal for benign diagnoses.[34] This controversy has been heightened by recent reports of trocar site recurrences of cancer in patients undergoing laparoscopic colectomy for adenocarcinoma of the colon.[40] All of these instances have been in patients who underwent laparoscopy with pneumoperitoneum, and recurrences have occurred at trocar sites, remote from the sites of colon specimen removal, in most cases. It is not known whether pneumoperitoneum is responsible for this high incidence of abdominal-wall recurrences.

Laparoscopic Appendectomy

Laparoscopic technique has proven more widely acceptable for performing appendectomy than for more complex abdominal procedures other than cholecystectomy. Laparoscopic appendectomy was first described in 1982 and predates the description of laparoscopic cholecystectomy.[41] However, the rapid and widespread acceptance of laparoscopic cholecystectomy coupled with the development of new and innovative laparoscopic instrumentation has sparked a renewed enthusiasm for laparoscopic appendectomy. Laparoscopic appendectomy can be readily applied with a high degree of success to a diverse group of patients presenting with acute appendicitis.[42]

Laparoscopic appendectomy is performed with the patient in the supine condition. The operating surgeon stands to the patient's right or between the patient's legs. Pneumoperitoneum is established through the umbilicus using the closed technique and the laparoscope is generally placed through the umbilicus. Additional ports are placed in the suprapubic area and in the right lower quadrant to facilitate dissection of the appendix (Figure 3.5).

Multiple randomized prospective comparisons of open versus laparoscopic appendectomy have appeared in the recent literature. Ortega and asso-

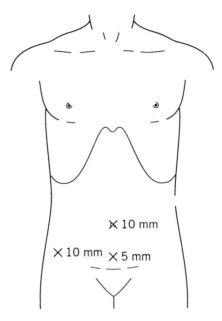

Figure 3.5. Laparoscopic appendectomy.

ciates reported a series of 253 patients randomized to one of the following groups: open appendectomy, laparoscopic appendectomy using the linear stapler, or laparoscopic appendectomy using catgut sutures.[43] Open appendectomy was performed with a statistically significant shorter duration of operation; however, wound infections were more common in patients undergoing open appendectomy. Patients undergoing laparoscopic appendectomy had shorter hospital stays, experienced less postoperative pain, and had a more rapid return to full activity.

Other studies have demonstrated that laparoscopic appendectomy requires longer operative times but shorter hospital stays.[43–46] The issue of postoperative pain has been found to be less or no different than in other studies. As more experience with laparoscopic appendectomy is gained, its place in the management of this common abdominal condition will become more clear.

Laparoscopic Splenectomy

Reports describing techniques for laparoscopic removal of the spleen first appeared in the literature in 1992.[47] Since that time several authors have described techniques for laparoscopic splenectomy using CO_2 pneumoperitoneum.[48-52] As with other laparoscopic operative techniques, a definite learning curve has been described, and operative times are longer than with open techniques; however, the benefits of minimal surgical access, less postoperative discomfort, and shorter hospital stays, are seen in patients who undergo these innovative procedures.[16,36]

Cadiere and associates perform laparoscopic splenectomy from an anterior abdominal approach with the patient in the supine position.[48] The surgeon stands between the patient's legs, and first and second assistants stand to the left and right sides of the patient, respectively. Five trocars are used and are positioned exactly as described for performing laparoscopic Nissen fundoplication.

Yee and coworkers also perform laparoscopic splenectomy with the patient in the supine lithotomy position with the surgeon standing between the patient's legs.[52] Four or five ports, placed similarly to the positioning used for laparoscopic Nissen fundoplication, are used to perform the operation.

Emmermann and associates[50] have recently reported an anterior abdominal technique for laparoscopic splenectomy where the surgeon and first assistant stand to the right side of the patient, the laparoscope is introduced through a supraumbilical incision, and the three operative ports are placed in a semicircular arrangement around the spleen. This technique was successful in 22 of 27 patients who underwent splenectomies by this approach for diagnoses of ITP, HIV, hairy cell leukemia, or for staging of Hodgkin's disease.

Hashizume and colleagues perform laparoscopic splenectomy with the patient in the right semidecubitus position and the surgeon standing on the patient's right side.[49] Pneumoperitoneum is established with the patient in the supine position through a 1-cm open incision in the left pararectal line above and to the left of the umbilicus. The laparoscope is introduced through this incision and the patient is then positioned in the right semidecubitus position for the operation. Three or four operative cannulae are placed in the left upper abdomen: one in the epigastric area, one in the mid-clavicular line of the left subcostal space, one in the mid-axillary line of the subcostal space, and optionally a fourth cannula in the lateral eighth intercostal space for patients with larger builds. These authors utilize the laparoscopic ultrasonic dissector to expose the splenic artery and vein and have reported successful application of this technique in four patients.

Delaitre utilizes a similar right semidecubitus position to perform his "hanged spleen" technique for laparoscopic splenectomy.[51] He utilizes five anteriorly placed trocars with pneumoperitoneum established through the standard umbilical route with a 10–12 mm cannula introduced at this site for placement of the laparoscope. A second cannula (5-mm) is placed to the right of the midline, between the ribs and umbilicus; a third cannulae (5-mm) is placed near the lower left ribs. A fourth cannula (5-mm) is inserted in the left paramedian-epigastric region. The final cannula (12-mm) is located between the umbilicus and the lower left rib for placement of the clip applier and the endo-GIA stapler.

III. COMPARISONS OF PNEUMOPERITONEUM VERSUS OPEN OPERATION

Physiologic and Operative Stress

Many comparisons of open versus laparoscopic operations have been made.[19,22,24,38,43–45,53–55] It has been generally established that laparoscopic abdominal procedures, where pneumoperitoneum is utilized, results in subjective improvements in patients' complaints of postoperative pain, and patients are able to leave the hospital sooner than those who undergo open operations.[56] A recent report by Senagore and coworkers indicates that patients who undergo laparoscopic-assisted colectomy, when compared to those who undergo open colectemy, resume enteral nutrition earlier with the result of earlier return to positive nitrogen balance.[54] The physiologic response to surgical stress in these patients was similar, as depicted by similar daily nitrogen losses in both groups; however, because those undergoing laparoscopic-assisted colectomy were able to resume enteral feedings earlier, they more quickly established positive nitrogen balance postoperatively.

Recently, Maruszynski and Pojda[57] demonstrated that surgical trauma, as detected by monitoring serum IL-6 levels for up to 72 hours postoperatively, in patients undergoing laparoscopy with pneumoperitoneum was less than that of patients undergoing open cholecystectomy. At all times postoperatively, the patients who underwent laparoscopic cholecystectomy had significantly lower serum IL-6 levels than those undergoing open cholecystectomy. IL-6 is a multifunctional cytokine involved in the modulation of the inflammatory process, and elevated levels of IL-6 correlate with increased surgical trauma and increased risk of postoperative complications. This study provides objective information that correlates with clinical observations of improved patient tolerance for laparoscopic procedures compared with open procedures.

In a more rigorous study of surgical-stress response, Glaser and colleagues demonstrated that patients undergoing laparoscopic cholecystectomy demonstrated less trauma and surgical stress than patients undergoing conventional cholecystectomy.[58] Postoperative epinephrine, norepinephrine, and glucose were consistently and significantly higher in patients undergoing conventional cholecystectomy. Norepinephrine, epinephrine, and glucose are all well-known markers of surgical stress and metabolic response to injury. Additionally, IL-6 expression was compared in these patients and found, as in the above study, to be significantly elevated in patients undergoing conventional cholecystectomy compared with laparoscopic cholecystectomy. Cortisol and ACTH responses were consistently, though not statistically, significant and lower in the laparoscopic versus the conventional cholecystectomy group.

Milheiro and associates[59] conducted a study of the metabolic responses to cholecystectomy. The study demonstrated no differences in postoperative serum cortisol or renin between patients undergoing open cholecystectomy or laparoscopic cholecystectomy. Serum values were measured serially over a 48-hour period postoperatively.

Postoperative Infections

Postoperative infection rates have been compared in patients undergoing laparoscopic and open abdominal procedures. These comparisons have been most meaningful in acute appendicitis, which carries a significant postoperative infection risk due to the inflammatory and infectious nature of the underlying process.

Ortega and coworkers, in a randomized prospective comparison of laparoscopic appendectomy with open appendectomy in 253 patients, demonstrated a significantly lower incidence of postoperative wound infections in patients undergoing laparoscopic appendectomy with the linear stapler and with catgut sutures when compared to patients undergoing open appendectomy.[43]

Kum and colleagues observed 109 patients in a randomized prospective study of open versus laparoscopic appendectomy (57 open, 52 laparoscopic).[60] The wound infection rate in the open group was 9% (5 patients) and 0% (0 patients) in the laparoscopic group ($p < 0.01$). Similar low rates of infection have been demonstrated in nonrandomized and retrospective comparisons of open versus laparoscopic appendectomy.[61,62]

The mechanisms of the reduced postoperative wound infection rates following laparoscopic procedures remain unclear. Trokel and associates demonstrated that immune responses to the immunogens keyhole limpet hemocyanine (KLH) and phytohemagluttin (PTH) were significantly diminished in rats undergoing open laparotomy, whereas the response to these immunogens was indistinguishable from control responses in rats undergoing CO_2 pneumoperitoneum.[63] This study suggests that immune competence is better preserved following pneumoperitoneum than after open laparotomy. Similar results have not been demonstrated in humans.

Miner and associates studied the growth of *Staphylococcus aureus* and *Escherichia coli* under atmospheric conditions similar to those of operative laparoscopy. They found that growth of these organisms was not suppressed by an atmospheric environment similar to that of CO_2 pneumoperitoneum and concluded that the laparoscopic atmosphere had no inhibitory effect on their growth.[64]

IV. SUMMARY AND CONCLUSIONS

Carbon dioxide pneumoperitoneum is the procedure of choice for performing laparoscopic abdominal operations. Laparoscopic cholecystectomy was the first procedure introduced into the routine armamentarium of the general surgeon and has allowed surgeons to become familiar with operating in two dimensions utilizing videoscopic equipment. Laparoscopic techniques have now been extended to include virtually every intraabdominal organ.[26,65–71] Surgeon acceptance of laparoscopic operations, other than cholecystectomy, has been slower due to the technical demands of advanced laparoscopic techniques.[33,36] Acceptance of these procedures has been hampered by deficiencies in laparoscopic instrumentation and the limitations imposed by the necessity of maintaining pneumoperitoneum during these procedures. Ongoing investigation is introducing newer methods into this burgeoning field that should make some of these procedures more acceptable to general surgeons.

Much has been made of the advantages of laparoscopic operations in terms of the reduced postoperative pain and morbidity patients experience following laparoscopic procedures. Most laparoscopic abdominal operations allow patients to resume normal activity sooner than they could after open abdominal operations. Compared with open procedures, there is a lower incidence of wound infection following laparoscopic abdominal operations and the biochemical stress response is more limited.[27,38,72,73]

Carbon-dioxide pneumoperitoneum is associated with known hemodynamic consequences and may be dangerous in patients with preexisting cardiopulmonary disease.[8] Carbon dioxide has been utilized for laparoscopic general surgical procedures because it is noncombustible, inexpensive, and readily absorbed. Other gases, such as helium and nitrous oxide, offer similar advantages to carbon dioxide and may have advantages that make them more attractive. Further research is necessary to ensure the safety of these agents for routine use in laparoscopy.

Caution must be exercised in applying laparoscopy to resection of abdominal malignancies due to the disturbing number of reports of trocar-site recurrences of colon and gallbladder cancers.[40,74] The incidence of these recurrences appear to be much higher than that reported for open operations. All of the reported cases were performed using pneumoperitoneum, but it is not known whether, or how, pneumoperitoneum may have contributed to these recurrences. Further investigation of this phenomenon is warranted prior to the widespread use of laparoscopy in abdominal cancer surgery.

Despite this warning, the field of laparoscopic abdominal surgery is growing rapidly. Reports of new and improved laparoscopic techniques appear monthly in the surgical literature. These new procedures must be evaluated with respect to the established standards of surgical practice, and must be held to these standards in terms of their utility and safety.[45] Much anticipation is warranted as this field continues to develop.

REFERENCES

1. Stellato TA: "History of laparoscopic surgery." Surg Clin North Am 1992, 72:997–1002.

2. Millard JA, Hill BB, Cook PS, et al.: "Intermittent sequential pneumatic compression in prevention of venous stasis associated with pneumoperitoneum during laparoscopic cholecystectomy." Arch Surg 1993, 128:914–918; discussion 918–919.

3. Wilson YG, Allen PE, Skidmore R, Baker AR: "Influence of compression stockings on lower-limb venous haemodynamics during laparoscopic cholecystectomy." Br J Surg 1994, 81:841–844.

4. Safran DB, Orlando R III: "Physiologic effects of pneumoperitoneum." Am J Surg 1994, 167:281–286.

5. Karatassas A, Walsh D, Hamilton DW: "A safe, new approach to establishing a pneumoperitoneum at laparoscopy." Aust N Z J Surg 1992, 62:489–491.

6. McKernan JB, Champion JK: "Access techniques: Veress needle—initial blind trocar insertion versus open laparoscopy with the Hasson trocar." Endosc Surg Allied Technol 1995, 3:35–38.

7. Byron JW, Markenson G, Miyazawa K: "A randomized comparison of Veress needle and direct trocar insertion for laparoscopy." Surg Gynecol Obstet 1993, 177:259–262.

8. Wolf JS, Clayman RV, Monk TG, et al.: "Carbon dioxide absorption during laparoscopic pelvic operation." J Am Coll Surg 1995, 180:555–560.

9. Wolf JS, Stoller ML: "The physiology of laparoscopy: basic principles, complications and other considerations." J Urol 1994, 152:294–302.

10. Windberger U, Siegl H, Ferguson JG, et al.: "Hemodynamic effects of prolonged abdominal insufflation for laparoscopic procedures." Gastrointest Endosc 1995, 41:121–129.

11. Leighton TA, Liu SY, Bongard FS: "Comparative cardiopulmonary effects of carbon dioxide versus helium pneumoperitoneum." Surgery 1993, 113:527–531.

12. Fredman B, Jedeikin R, Olsfanger D, et al.: "Residual pneumoperitoneum: a cause of postoperative pain after laparoscopic cholecystectomy." Anesth Analg 1994, 79:152–154.

13. Hunter JG, Staheli J, Oddsdottir M, Trus T: "Nitrous oxide pneumoperitoneum revisited: Is there a risk of combustion? Surg Endosc 1995, 9:501–504.

14. Rademaker BM, Odoom JA, de Wit LT, et al.: "Haemodynamic effects of pneumoperitoneum for laparoscopic surgery: a comparison of CO$_2$ and N$_2$O insufflation." Eur J Anaesthesiol 1994, 11:301–306.

15. Callery MP, Soper NJ: "Physiology of the pneumoperitoneum." Baillieres Clin Gastroenterol 1993, 7:757–777.

16. Moore MJ, Bennett CL: "The learning curve for laparoscopic cholecystectomy. The Southern Surgeons Club." Am J Surg 1995, 170:55–59.

17. Meyers WC: "The Southern Surgeons Club: A Prospective Analysis of 1518 Laparoscopic Cholecystectomies." N Engl J Med 1991, 324:1073–1078.

18. Reddick EJ, Olsen DO: "Laparoscopic laser cholecystectomy. A comparison with mini-lap cholecystectomy." Surg Endosc 1989, 3:131–133.

19. Kane RL, Lurie N, Borbas C, et al.: "The outcomes of elective laparoscopic and open cholecystectomies [see comments]." J Am Coll Surg 1995, 180:136–145.

20. Nowzaradan Y, Barnes P: "Laparoscopic Nissen fundoplication." J Laparoendosc Surg 1993, 3:429–438.

21. Bittner HB, Meyers WC, Brazer SR, Pappas TN: "Laparoscopic Nissen fundoplication: operative results and short-term follow-up." Am J Surg 1994, 167:193–198; discussion 199–220.

22. Rattner DW, Brooks DC: "Patient satisfaction following laparoscopic and open antireflux surgery." Arch Surg 1995, 130:289–293; discussion 293–294.

23. Cuschieri A, Shimi S, Nathanson LK: "Laparoscopic reduction, crural repair, and fundoplication of large hiatal hernia." Am J Surg 1992, 163:425–430.

24. Peters JH, Heimbucher J, Kauer WK, et al.: "Clinical and physiologic comparison of laparoscopic and open Nissen fundoplication." J Am Coll Surg 1995, 180:385–393.

25. McKernan JB, Wolfe BM, MacFadyen BV: "Laparoscopic repair of duodenal ulcer and gastroesophageal reflux." Surg Clin North Am 1992, 72:1153–1167.

26. Fontaumard E, Espalieu P, Boulez J: "Laparoscopic Nissen-Rossetti fundoplication: first results." Surg Endosc 1995, 9:869–873.

27. Snow LL, Weinstein LS, Hannon JK: "Laparoscopic reconstruction of gastroesophageal anatomy for the treatment of reflux disease." Surg Endosc 1995, 9:774–780.

28. Rosati R, Fumagalli U, Bonavina L, et al.: "Laparoscopic approach to esophageal achalasia." Am J Surg 1995, 169:424–427.

29. Oddsdottir M, Franco AL, Laycock WS, et al.: "Laparoscopic repair of paraesophageal hernia. New access, old technique." Surg Endosc 1995, 9:164–168.

30. Pitcher DE, Curet MJ, Martin DT, et al.: "Successful laparoscopic repair of paraesophageal hernia." Arch Surg 1995, 130:590–596.

31. Beart RW: "Laparoscopic colectomy: Status of the art." Dis Colon Rectum 1994, 37:S47–S49.

32. Sackier JM, Slutzki S, Wood C, et al.: "Laparoscopic endocorporeal mobilization followed by extracorporeal sutureless anastomosis for the treatment of carcinoma of the left colon." Dis Colon Rectum 1993, 36:610–612.

33. Sosa JL, Sleeman D, Puente I, et al.: "Laparoscopic-assisted colostomy closure after Hartmann's procedure." Dis Colon Rectum 1994, 37:149–152.

34. Franklin ME, Rosenthal D, Norem RF: "Prospective evaluation of laparoscopic colon resection versus open colon resection for adenocarcinoma: A multicenter study." Surg Endosc 1995, 9:811–816.

35. Reissman P, Teoh TA, Piccirillo M, et al.: "Colonoscopic-assisted laparoscopic colectomy." Surg Endosc 1994, 8:1352–1353.

36. Simons AJ, Anthone GJ, Ortega AE, et al.: "Laparoscopic-assisted colectomy learning curve." Dis Colon Rectum 1995, 38:600–603.

37. Ramos JM, Beart RW, Goes R, et al.: "Role of laparoscopy in colorectal surgery. A prospective evaluation of 200 cases." Dis Colon Rectum 1995, 38:494–501.

38. Wexner SD, Johansen OB, Nogueras JJ, Jagelman DG: "Laparoscopic total abdominal colectomy. A prospective trial." Dis Colon Rectum 1992, 35:651–655.

39. Elftmann TD, Nelson H, Ota DM, et al.: "Laparoscopic-assisted segmental colectomy: surgical techniques." Mayo Clin Proc 1994, 69:825–833.

40. Cirocco WC, Schwartzman A, Golub RW: "Abdominal wall recurrence after laparoscopic colectomy for colon cancer." Surgery 1994, 116:842–846.

41. Semm K: "Endoskopische Methoden in Gastroenterologie und Gynakologie. Erganzung der diagnostischen Peviskopie durch die endoskopische Abdominalchirurgie. [Endoscopic methods in gastroenterology and gynecology. Completion of diagnostic pelviscopy by endoscopic abdominal surgery]" Fortschr Med 1984, 102:534–537.

42. Pier A, Gotz F, Bacher C: "Laparoscopic appendectomy in 625 cases: from innovation to routine." Surg Laparosc Endosc 1991, 1:8–13.

43. Ortega AE, Hunter JG, Peters JH, et al.: "A prospective, randomized comparison of laparoscopic appendectomy with open appendectomy. Laparoscopic Appendectomy Study Group." Am J Surg 1995, 169:208–212; discussion 212–213.

44. Bonanni F, Reed JE, Hartzell G, et al.: "Laparoscopic versus conventional appendectomy." J Am Coll Surg 1994, 179:273–278.

45. Heinzelmann M, Simmen HP, Cummins AS, Largiader F: "Is laparoscopic appendectomy the new 'gold standard'?" Arch Surg 1995, 130:782–785.

46. MacFayden BV, Wolfe BM, McKernan JB: "Laparoscopic management of the acute abdomen, appendix, and small and large bowel." Surg Clin North Am 1992, 72:1169–1183.

47. Rhodes M, Rudd M, O'Rourke N, et al.: "Laparoscopic splenectomy and lymph node biopsy for hematologic disorders." Ann Surg 1995, 222:43–46.

48. Cadiere GB, Verroken R, Himpens J, et al.: "Operative strategy in laparoscopic splenectomy." J Am Coll Surg 1994, 179:668–672.

49. Hashizume M, Sugimachi K. Kitano S, et al.: "Laparoscopic splenectomy." Am J Surg 1994, 167:611–614.

50. Emmermann A, Zornig C, Peiper M, et al.: "Laparoscopic Splenectomy: technique and results in a series of 27 cases." Surg Endosc 1995, 9:924–927.

51. Delaitre B: "Laparoscopic splenectomy: The "hanged spleen" technique." Surg Endosc 1995, 9:528–529.

52. Yee LF, Carvajal SH, deLorimer AA, Mulvihill SJ: "Laparoscopic Splenectomy: The initial experience at University of California, San Francisco." Arch Surg 1995, 130:874–879.

53. Prinz RA: "A comparison of laparoscopic and open adrenalectomies." Arch Surg 1995, 130:489–492; discussion 492–494.

54. Senagore AJ, Kilbride MJ, Luchtefeld MA, et al.: "Superior nitrogen balance after laparoscopic-assisted colectomy." Ann Surg 1995, 221:171–175.

55. Harmon GD, Senagore AJ, Kilbride MJ, Warzynski MJ: "Interleukin-6 response to laparoscopic and open colectomy." Dis Colon Rectum 1994, 37:754–759.

56. Ballantyne GH: "Laparoscopic-assisted colorectal surgery: Review of results in 752 patients." Gastroenterologist 1995, 3:75–89.

57. Maruszynski M, Pojda Z: "Interleukin 6 (IL-6) levels in the monitoring of surgical trauma: a comparison of serum IL-6 concentrations in patients treated by cholecystectomy via laparotomy or laparoscopy." Surg Endosc 1995, 9:882–885.

58. Glaser F, Sannwald GA, Buhr HJ, et al.: "General stress response to conventional and laparoscopic cholecystectomy." Ann Surg 1995, 221:372–380.

59. Milheiro A, Sousa FC, Manso EC, Leitao F: "Metabolic responses to cholecystectomy: open vs. laparoscopic approach." J Laparoendosc Surg 1994, 4:311–317.

60. Kum CK, Ngoi SS, Goh PM, et al.: "Randomized controlled trial comparing laparoscopic and open appendicectomy." Br J Surg 1993, 80:1599–1600.

61. Lujan Mompean JA, Robles Campos R, et al.: "Laparoscopic versus open appendicectomy: a prospective assessment." Br J Surg 1994, 81:133–135.

62. McAnena OJ, Austin O, O'Connell PR, et al.: "Laparoscopic versus open appendicectomy: A prospective evaluation." Br J Surg 1992, 79:818–820.

63. Trokel MJ, Bessler M, Treat MR, et al.: "Preservation of immune response after laparoscopy." Surg Endosc 1994, 8:1385–1387; discussion 1387–1388.

64. Miner DW, Levine RL: "Microbiologic effects of atmospheric conditions used in operative laparoscopy." J. Reprod Med 1993, 38:531–533.

65. Anvari M, Park A: "Laparoscopic-assisted vagotomy and distal gastrectomy." Surg Endosc 1994, 8:1312–1315.

66. Arnaud JP, Casa C, Manunta A: "Laparoscopic continent gastrostomy." Am J Surg 1995, 169:629–630.

67. Curet MJ, Pitcher DE, Martin DT, Zucker KA: "Laparoscopic antegrade sphincterotomy. A new technique for the management of complex choledocholithiasis." Ann Surg 1995, 221:149–155.

68. Fernandez-Cruz L, Saenz A, Benarroch G, et al.: "Technical aspects of adrenalectomy via operative laparoscopy." Surg Endosc 1994, 8:1348–1351.

69. Avrahami R, Watemberg S, Hiss Y, Deutsch AA: "Laparoscopic vs conventional autopsy. A promising perspective." Arch Surg 1995, 130:407–409.

70. Hunter JG: "Laparoscopic transcystic common bile duct exploration." Am J Surg 1992, 163:53–56; discussion 57–58.

71. Senagore AJ, Kilbride MJ, Luchtefeld MA, et al.: "Superior nitrogen balance after laparoscopic-assisted colectomy." Ann Surg 1995, 221:171–175.

72. Bohm B, Milsom JW, Fazio VW: "Postoperative intestinal motility following conventional and laparoscopic intestinal surgery." Arch Surg 1995, 130:415–519.

73. Fischer JE: "The metabolic response to laparoscopic cholecystectomy [editorial]." Ann Surg 1995, 221:211–213.

74. Fong Y, Brennan MF, Turnbull A, et al.: "Gallbladder cancer discovered during laparoscopic surgery. Potential for iatrogenic tumor dissemination [see comments]." Arch Surg 1993, 128:1054–1056.

4

LOW-PRESSURE PNEUMOPERITONEUM

David M. Brams, M.D.
Edmund K. M. Tsoi, M.S., M.D.
Jay K. Harness, M.D.

I. INTRODUCTION

The development of videolaparoscopy in conjunction with pneumoperitoneum has revolutionized the field of general surgery. Pneumoperitoneum distends the abdominal cavity and provides the surgeon with excellent exposure in a working space that is visualized by the videoscopic laparoscope. However, pneumoperitoneum also has deleterious effects at higher pressures.[1–2] The occurrence of complications associated with high intraabdominal pressure has led to the acceptance of a standard insufflation pressure of 15 mm Hg, which allows good visualization with minimal cardiopulmonary complications.

Certain patients poorly tolerate intraabdominal pressures of 15 mm Hg: those who have cardiac or pulmonary disease, those who are hypovolemic sec-

Abdominal Access in Open and Laparoscopic Surgery
Edited by Edmund K. M. Tsoi and Claude H. Organ, Jr.
ISBN 0-471-13352-3 Copyright © 1996 by Wiley-Liss, Inc.

ondary to trauma or critical illness, and those who are awake. In these patients, a lower intraabdominal pressure is needed.

The use of low-pressure pneumoperitoneum is not well documented because most patients tolerate 15 mm Hg of pressure. In this chapter we will discuss the potential advantages of low-pressure pneumoperitoneum and situations in which its use is preferred.

II. A HISTORICAL PERSPECTIVE: WHY 15 mm Hg?

The use of pneumoperitoneum was first proposed by Otto Goetze of Germany in 1918.[3] He suggested that an insufflation needle originally intended for diagnostic radiology could be used for laparoscopy. The insufflation needle with a shielded top was introduced in 1917 by Janos Veress of Hungary and was used for the drainage of pleural effusion and ascites. This same needle was used to gain access to the peritoneum for laparoscopy with the insufflation of gas.[4] In 1924, Zollikofer of Switzerland suggested using carbon dioxide for insufflation, thus obviating the potential hazards of explosion encountered with oxygen pneumoperitoneum and allowing the benefits associated with the rapid absorption of carbon dioxide.[5]

Laparoscopists initially used high intraabdominal pressures; however, complications associated with pressures greater than 30 mm Hg led to a search for a standard pressure that optimized visualization and at the same time minimized cardiopulmonary complications. Surgeons found that the abdominal cavity could be fully distended with pneumoperitoneal pressure between 15 and 20 mm Hg. Prior to the development of videolaparoscopy, several studies in the gynecologic and anesthesia literature noted the deleterious effects of pneumoperitoneum with carbon dioxide at these pressures. It was noted that in patients undergoing pelvic laparoscopy there was a significant fall in arterial pH, a rise in arterial pCO_2, and a rise in airway pressures required to maintain a constant volume of ventilation.[6-7]

Alexander et al. suggested that these changes were due to CO_2 absorption across the peritoneum.[8] More recently, Ho and his colleagues demonstrated in the animal model that carbon dioxide used during laparoscopy results in systemic carbon-dioxide absorption across the peritoneum, leading to hypercapnia, acidosis, and depressed hemodynamics.[9-10] In normovolemic patients, the deleterious effects were limited with pressures less than 25 mm Hg in the absence of severe cardiopulmonary disease.[11] Recently, McDougall and associates demonstrated that 94% of the abdominal volume is achieved by CO_2 insufflation to 15 mm Hg. Furthermore, the force of insertion of various mechanical trocars is not significantly different between insufflation to a pressure of 15 mm Hg versus 30 mm Hg.[12]

In most patients, as pneumoperitoneum increases to 25 mm Hg, blood pressure, central venous pressure, and cardiac output all rise. This is probably related to increased sympathetic tone secondary to hypercarbia. As intraabdominal pressure continues to rise to 40 mm Hg, blood pressure, central venous pressure, and cardiac output all drop. This occurs due to mechanical compression of the intraabdominal vena cava as well as the effects of carbon dioxide retention, which include acidosis and direct negative inotropic effects.[13] These effects are rarely seen in the intubated patient who is mechanically ventilated and is not hypovolemic. In patients with preexisting pulmonary disease, there is an increase in end-tidal carbon dioxide with acidosis. Increased minute ventilation may help excrete this, although perhaps at the risk of barotrauma.[14] Furthermore, increased intrathoracic pressures resulting from increased ventilation may also impair venous return. Ho et al. have demonstrated in the animal model that 15 mm Hg intraabdominal pressure has no adverse effect on either hemodynamics or metabolic function. However, in the setting of hemorrhagic shock, there is hemodynamic depression due to both the potentiated effects of hypercapnia as well as the increased intraabdominal pressure impairing venous return.[15]

One strategy used to avoid these complications is to decrease insufflation pressures. Jorgensen and colleagues examined lower-limb venous hemodynamics in pigs during laparoscopy to assess the impact of raised intraabdominal pressures on femoral venous outflow. Their experimental animal model demonstrated a profound decrease in femoral venous blood flow as intraabdominal pressure increased above 10 mm Hg.[16] Studies done at the Department of Surgery at the University of California–Davis, East Bay by Tsoi and associates have demonstrated that laparoscopic procedures can be safely performed using low-pressure pneumoperitoneum (< 11 mm Hg) and at the same time cause less impediment of venous blood flow in the femoral vein.[17] The University of California researchers have also noted that the distance between the abdominal wall and the abdominal viscera is smaller with low-pressure pneumoperitoneum than with the standard 15 mm Hg of pressure. There-fore, extra care should be taken in trocar placement. Low-pressure pneu-moperitoneum can be used in patients who are not mechanically ventilated, who have poor pulmonary function, who are critically ill and hypovolemic, and who are pregnant.

III. LOW-PRESSURE PNEUMOPERITONEUM LAPAROSCOPY

We prefer the use of low-pressure laparoscopy (less than 12 mm Hg) in several settings. Diagnostic laparoscopy in the awake patient can be performed readi-ly using local anesthesia and low intraabdominal pressure. Videoscopic enter-al-access procedures are also facilitated using low pressures that allow the ab-dominal wall to be approximated to the stomach or small bowel. In addition, diagnostic minilaparoscopy can be accomplished in the awake trauma patient. Finally, exposure obtained with low-pressure laparoscopy can be augmented with mechanical lifting devices.

IV. DIAGNOSTIC LAPAROSCOPY UNDER LOCAL ANESTHESIA

In 1937 Ruddock, an internist, published his experience using local anesthesia to perform 500 cases of peritoneoscopy.[18] Despite his success, laparoscopy tra-ditionally was still performed under general anesthesia. Although most la-paroscopic procedures are today performed under general anesthesia with 15 mm Hg of CO_2 pneumoperitoneum, there are advocates for performing la-paroscopy with a lower pressure and local anesthesia.

   In 1992 Childers and his colleagues reported the use of a fiberoptic catheter (1.8 mm in diameter) to perform laparoscopy and biopsy.[19] Six of the seven patients had their laparoscopic procedure done in their physician's of-fice. Local anesthesia together with intravenous sedation and low-pressure pneumoperitoneum (< 15 mm Hg) were used in all seven cases. Salkey has used local anesthesia and nitrous-oxide (N_2O) insufflation pressures of 10–12 mm Hg to examine patients with abdominal pain, focal liver disease, abdominal mass, ascites of unknown etiology, and to perform prelaparotomy and second-look procedures.[20] The advantages of local anesthesia include avoiding the risks of general anesthesia and being able to localize areas of pain with patient cooperation. Nitrous oxide is used to avoid the peritoneal irritation associated with carbon dioxide; hypercapnia and its effects are also avoided. Salkey recommends that laparoscopy be performed in the operating room with the patient mildly sedated. Intravenous injection of a short-acting benzodiazapine, such as midazolam, is preferred. The skin and subcutaneous tissues are thoroughly anesthetized using 0.25 percent bupivicaine. Epinephrine is avoided due to the systemic effects it occasionally causes. The peritoneum is also infiltrated with a local anesthetic. The initial puncture site is made in the supraumbilical position. A site 2.5 cm lateral from the midline traversing the rectus yet avoiding the inferior epigastric vessels is used for Veress-needle placement. The umbilical region should be avoided in patients with portal hypertension and abdominal wall collaterals. In patients with ascites, a camera port site is placed more cephalad in order to reach the hepatic space during laparoscopic exploration.

Salkey has described his "push out" technique, which he uses in patients who have not previously undergone abdominal surgery. The technique is so named because these patients "push out" their abdominal-wall musculature in resistance to the insertion of instruments. In cases of prior abdominal operation, an open technique can be used. After confirmation of the intraabdominal location of the needle using the saline drop test, N_2O insufflation is performed at a slow rate (1 L/min). When an intraabdominal pressure of 10 mm Hg is reached, a 5- or 10-mm trocar can be inserted to allow visualization with the laparoscope. Additional trocars can be inserted after tissues have been anesthetized.

Salkey performed 780 diagnostic procedures, 93% of which were completed successfully using local anesthesia. The only complication he encountered was one episode of reflex bradycardia. He found adequate visualization using low-pressure pneumoperitoneum and his experience demonstrates that the judicious use of this technique allows abdominal exploration to be performed under local anesthesia with a minimum of complications. The increased use of the miniature optical catheter will undoubtedly allow the surgeon to perform more laparoscopy in an outpatient facility using local anesthesia with low-pressure pneumoperitoneum.

V. VIDEOSCOPICALLY GUIDED ENTERAL ACCESS

Since the introduction of videolaparoscopy, there have been several reports of the use of laparoscopic gastrostomy and jejunostomy as alternatives to the open technique in settings precluding endoscopic placement of enteral-access catheters.[21-25] These procedures are performed with a low-pressure pneumoperitoneum that allows the viscous organ to be approximated to the abdominal wall. Laparoscopic gastrostomy is indicated in patients for whom percutaneous endoscopic gastrostomy (PEG) is not possible due to esophageal obstruction or severe obesity that limits abdominal-wall transillumination, and in patients who require gastrostomy and are undergoing laparoscopy for other reasons (Table 4.1). Patients who have had prior surgery and who have multiple adhesions that preclude PEG can be a candidate for laparoscopic surgery.

In 1993 Duh and Way described their method for performing gastrostomy and jejunostomy. Either general or local anesthesia was employed. If possible, a nasogastric tube was placed to deflate the stomach. A Veress-needle or open technique was then used to gain access to the stomach. The intraabdominal pressure was reduced to between 6 and 10 mm Hg. Duh and Way have used T-fasteners to secure the distended stomach or jejunum to the abdominal wall (Figure 4.1). These fasteners are metal T-bars attached to a nylon suture and then inserted into the bowel with a slotted needle. Using serial dilators, an 18-French balloon-tipped catheter was then placed into the stomach or jejunum over a guide wire. Using this technique, Duh placed 56 gastrostomy and jejunostomy tubes laparoscopically. There were no conversions to open procedures, only two complications, and no mortality related to catheter placement.[22-25]

Sylvester and associates have described the use of a microendoscope

TABLE 4.1

Indications for laparoscopic-assisted enteral access

Head and neck cancer
Esophageal cancer or obstruction
Morbid obesity
Previous abdominal surgery
Concomitant laparoscopic procedures

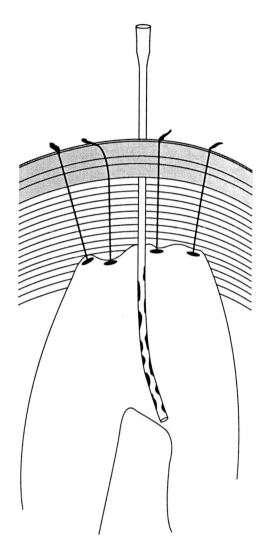

Figure 4.1. T-fastener holding bowel against abdominal wall.

placed through a specially designed Veress needle to directly visualize the stomach during PEG and thus avoid possible complications associated with this procedure.[26] After transillumination of the abdominal wall with the endoscope, the stomach is deflated and the special Veress needle is inserted. Only 500–800 cc of CO_2 are insufflated to a pressure of 4–5 mm Hg. Sylvester and his colleagues found that their patients tolerate this degree of abdominal pressure without difficulty. The central stylet of the Veress needle is then removed and a

1.7-mm "minilaparoscope" is inserted (Figure 4.2). After exploration of the upper abdomen, PEG is performed under direct vision in the usual fashion. Sylvester performed this combined procedure without morbidity or mortality in 10 of 11 consecutive patients. The single instance in which this procedure was not successful was due to equipment failure.[26]

Low-pressure pneumoperitoneum allows the abdominal wall to be approximated to the stomach or jejunum while also providing adequate exposure for catheter placement. Both of these techniques allow a minimally invasive approach to enteral access without the morbidity caused by an open procedure, the risks of PEG, and/or the standard pressures of pneumoperitoneum.

VI. LOW-PRESSURE LAPAROSCOPY IN THE EVALUATION OF TRAUMA

The use of laparoscopy in the evaluation of the trauma patient was first described by Lamy in 1956 in two patients with splenic trauma who were treated conservatively.[27] Since this article was published, there have been numerous reports of the use of laparoscopy in trauma. Although most diagnostic laparoscopy is done in the operating room under general anesthesia, there is a

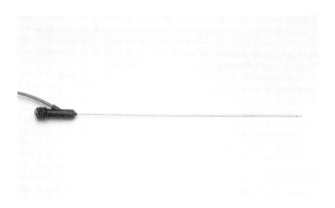

Figure 4.2. Minilaparoscope (courtesy of Origin Medsystem Inc., Menlo Park, California).

role for the use of videolaparoscopy in the emergency department using local anesthesia and low-pressure pneumoperitoneum.

In 1983 Berci et al. reported their experience with 106 patients with blunt abdominal trauma. They evaluated these patients in the emergency department (ED) with a 5-mm laparoscope inserted under local anesthesia. Their results suggested that laparoscopy was superior to diagnostic peritoneal lavage in that it provided a more accurate assessment of hemorrhage and whether or not laparotomy was required.[28]

In 1988 Cuschieri reported a randomized prospective multicenter trial comparing diagnostic laparoscopy with diagnostic peritoneal lavage (DPL). DPL led to nontherapeutic laparotomy in 3 of 11 patients versus only 1 of 13 patients in which laparoscopy was performed.[29] These results indicated that laparoscopy was as sensitive as and more selective than DPL.

Salvino and associates described their experience with 75 patients with blunt and penetrating trauma.[30] Ninety-three percent of the procedures were performed in the ED and 59% were performed under local anesthesia. All patients underwent laparoscopy followed by DPL. If DPL was positive, or if the laparoscopy was abnormal, the patient underwent laparotomy. Salvino and his colleagues found that laparoscopy would have improved care in 8% of the cases. They found laparoscopy to be more sensitive in cases of diaphragmatic injury (Figure 4.3).

Diagnostic laparoscopy is difficult to perform in the emergency department and should be performed only if a dedicated space and equipment are available. The patient must be fully monitored. The primary indication for diagnostic laparoscopy is to evaluate the patient for peritoneal penetration secondary to stab wounds or tangential gunshot wounds. Patients must be hemodynamically stable. To perform the procedure, the skin is infiltrated with local anesthesia and using either a Veress-needle or open technique a 5-mm port can be introduced. Eight to 10 mm Hg of N_2O is insufflated. A 5-mm laparoscope can then be used to explore the abdomen. Smaller laparoscopes (< 2 mm) that can be introduced through the Veress needle are also being developed.

Diagnostic laparoscopy allows the trauma surgeon to decide if there is peritoneal penetration or if there is significant injury due to blunt trauma. This information can then be used to triage the patient to observation, discharge, or to the operating room for complete laparoscopy or laparotomy.

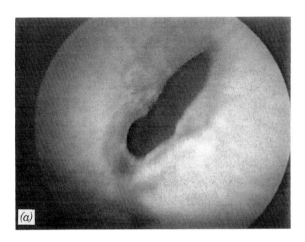

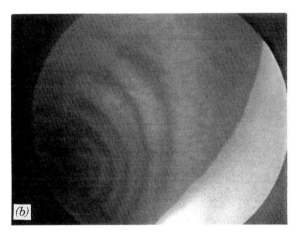

Figure 4.3. (*a*) Diaphragmatic laceration seen during trauma laparoscopy (courtesy of E. K. M. Tsoi). (*b*) Laparoscopic view of the thoracic cavity through the diaphragmatic laceration. (See insert for color representation.)

VII. OTHER REPORTED USES OF PNEUMOPERITONEUM

There have been many reports of other uses of low-pressure pneumoperitoneum. Kuster et al. described the repair of a diaphragmatic foramen-of-Morgagni hernia using a laparoscopic technique and CO_2 insufflation of 8 mm Hg.[31] Yamashita and his colleagues have performed laparoscopic resection of gastric leiomyoma using less than 8 mm Hg intraabdominal pressure.[32] Pendurthi et al. have even performed bilateral inguinal hernia repair under local anesthesia with low N_2O insufflation pressure (< 12 mm Hg).[33]

VIII. COMBINED METHODS

The complications associated with 15-mm Hg pneumoperitoneum as well as the limited exposure low-pressure pneumoperitoneum provides led to the development of adjunctive abdominal-wall lifting devices to augment the exposure afforded by this technique. In 1991 Gazayerli described an instrument to be inserted through a port; this instrument was then deployed into a T-shaped configuration.[34] A similar T-shaped abdominal-wall lifting device that connects to a telescoping stand mounted on the operating room table is now commercially available (Figure 4.4). This T-shaped retractor can elevate a portion of the abdominal wall to facilitate exposure. It was suggested for use in herniorrhaphy, in the obese, and in patients with marginal cardiopulmonary status.

In 1993 Banting and Cuschieri introduced their falciform lift. This instrument is a large curved trocar, 4 mm in diameter, to which is attached a flexible polyethylene tube 80 cm in length. After achieving 8 mm Hg of pneumoperitoneum and placement of a periumbilical port, this curved trocar is inserted through a stab wound in the left upper quadrant lateral to the falciform ligament. Under direct visualization, the trocar is passed through the abdomen around the falciform ligament and then exits to the right of the falciform ligament (Figure 4.5). The tubing is then suspended to a horizontal bar at the head of the operating room table by a hook-and-chain assembly. Banting et al. employed this technique in 12 patients with cardiac or pulmonary disease and achieved excellent visualization without complications.[35]

Inoue et al. described an abdominal-wall lifter using a flexible vinyl tube wall retractor, similar in design to that of Banting and his colleagues, yet placed from the super supraumbilical to the right upper abdominal area (Figure 4.5). They found that with their retractor they were able to achieve exposure with 10 mm Hg similar to that which occurs with pure pneumoperitoneum at 15 mm Hg of pressure.[36]

Go and colleagues reported on their experiences with laparoscopic

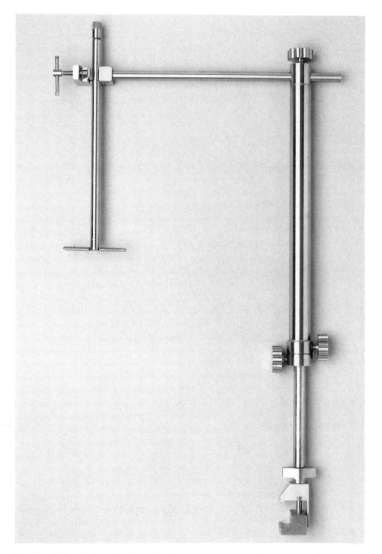

Figure 4.4. Bookler abdominal-wall-elevator retractor (courtesy of Mediflex Surgical Products, Islandia, New York).

adrenalectomy using low-pressure pneumoperitoneum in combination with abdominal-wall lifting by Kuntscher wire. They performed fourteen adrenalectomies for functioning adrenal lesions. These patients were positioned in a semidecubitus position. Pneumoperitoneal pressure of 12 mm Hg was used and five trocars were placed for the procedure. A Kuntscher-wire retractor was

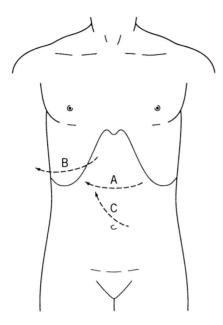

Figure 4.5. Diagram demonstrating the placement of flexible tubing or wire in combination with low-pressure pneumoperitoneum. (A) Banting et al.,[35] (B) Inoue et al.,[36] (C) Go et al.[37]

then placed subcutaneously in the right subcostal region (Figure 4.5) and retracted proximally, achieving excellent visualization with only 8 mm Hg of insufflation pressure.[37]

IX. CONCLUSIONS

Low-pressure pneumoperitoneum has a role in laparoscopy in critically ill patients, patients with cardiopulmonary problems, and pregnant patients. For certain tasks it provides adequate exposure without the deleterious effects of standard pneumoperitoneum. Low-pressure pneumoperitoneum could allow laparoscopy to be performed in patients who might otherwise not be able to tolerate the procedure. Using N_2O at lower pressures, the awake patient can also be evaluated in the setting of trauma or chronic disease. Diagnostic laparoscopy can also be done under local anesthesia in the office. Abdominal-wall retractors can augment the usefulness of low-pressure pneumoperitoneum, improve exposure without the detrimental effects of higher pressures, and be especially useful in complicated procedures where longer operating time is required.

REFERENCES

1. Richardson JD, Trinkle JK: "Hemodynamic and respiratory alterations with increased intra-abdominal pressure." J Surg Res 1976, 20:401–404.

2. Caldwell CB, Ricotta JJ: "Changes in visceral blood flow with elevated intra-abdominal pressure." J Surg Res 1987, 43:14–20.

3. Goetze O: "Die Roentgendiagnostik bei gasgefullter Bauchhohle: Eine neue Methode." Munch Med Wschr 1918, 65:12575–1280.

4. Veress J: "Neues Instrument zur Ausfuhrung von Brust- oder Bauchfunktionen und Pneumothorax behandlung." Dtsch Med Wschr 1938, 41:1480–1481.

5. Zollikofer R: "Zur Laparoskopie." Schweiz Med Wschr 1924, 54:84–87.

6. Hodgson C, McClelland RMA, Newton JR: "Some effects of the peritoneal insufflation of carbon dioxide at laparoscopy." Anesthesia 1970, 25:382–390.

7. Smith, I, Benzie RJ, Nanette LM, et al.: "Cardiovascular effects of peritoneal insufflation of carbon dioxide for laparoscopy." Br Med J 1971, 3:410–411.

8. Alexander G, Brown E: "Physiologic alternations during pelvic laparoscopy." Am J Obst Gynec 1969, 105:1078–1081.

9. Ho HS, Gunther RA, Wolfe BM: "Intraperitoneal carbon dioxide insufflation and cardiopulmonary functions." Arch Surg 1992, 127:928–933.

10. Ho HS, Saunders CJ, Wolfe BM: "Effector of hemodynamics during laparoscopy: CO_2 absorption or intra-abdominal pressure." University of California–Davis. Postgraduate Course.

11. Liu SY, Leighton T, Davis I, et al.: "Prospective analysis of cardiopulmonary responses to laparoscopic cholecystectomy." J Laparoendosc Surg 1991, 1:241–246.

12. McDougall EM, Figenshau RS, Clayman RV, et al.: "Laparoscopic pneumoperitoneum: Impact of body habitus." J Laparoendosc Surg 1994, 4:385–391.

13. Diamant M, Benumof JL, Saidman LJ: "Hemodynamics of increased intra-abdominal pressure: interaction with hypovolemia and halothane anesthesia." Anesthesiology 1978, 48:23–27.

14. Wittgen CM, Andrus CH, Fitzgerald SD, et al.: "Analysis of hemodynamic and ventilatory effect of laparoscopic cholecystectomy." Arch Surg 1991, 126:997–1001.

15. Ho HS, Eisenhauer DM, Wolfe BM: "Hemodynamic effects of N_2 pneumoperitoneum in hemorrhage." Surg Endosc 1994, 8:251 (Abstract).

16. Jorgensen JO, Gillies RB, Lalak NJ, et al.: "Lower limb venous hemodynamics during laparoscopy: An animal study." Surg Laparosc Endosc 1994, 4:32–35.

17. Tsoi EKM, Brams D, Goldstein LJ, unpublished data.

18. Ruddock EJ: "Peritoneoscopy." S G & O 1937, 65:623–639.

19. Childers JM, Hatch KD, Surwit EA: "Office laparoscopy and biopsy for evaluation of patients with intraperitoneal carcinomatosis using a new optical catheter." Gynecologic Oncology 1992, 47:337–342.

20. Salkey BA: "Local anesthesia in laparoscopy," Principles of Laparoscopic Surgery New York: Springer-Verlag, 1995, 87–90.

21. Reiner DS, Leitman IM, Ward RJ: "Laparoscopic Stamm gastrostomy with gastropexy." Surg Laparosc Endosc 1991, 1:189–192.

22. Duh QY, Way LW: "Laparoscopic jejunostomy using T-fasteners as retractors and anchors." Arch Surg 1993, 128:105–108.

23. Duh QY, Way LW: "Laparoscopic gastrostomy using T-fasteners as retractors and anchors." Surg Endosc 1993, 7:60–63.

24. Duh QY, Senokozlieff-Englehart AL, Siperstein AE, et al.: "Prospective evaluation of the safety and efficacy of laparoscopic jejunostomy." West J Med 1995, 162:117–122.

25. Duh QY: "Laparoscopic gastrostomy and jejunostomy." Surgical Rounds 1995, 18:143–151.

26. Sylvester KG, Paskin DL, Schuricht AL: "Combined laparoscopic-endoscopic gastrostomy." Surg Endosc 1994, 8:1072–1075.

27. Lamy J, Sarles H: "Intérêt de la péritonéoscopie chez les polytraumatises." Marseille Chir 1956, 8:82–86.

28. Berci G, Dunkelman D, Michel SL, et al.: "Emergency minilaparoscopy in abdominal trauma: An update." Am J Surg 1983, 146:261–265.

29. Cuschieri A, Hennessy TPJ, Stephens RB, et al.: "Diagnosis of significant abdominal trauma after road traffic accidents: Preliminary results of a multicentre clinical trial comparing minilaparoscopy with peritoneal lavage." Ann R Coll Surg (England) 1988, 70:153–155.

30. Salvino CK, Esposito TJ, Marshall WJ: "The role of diagnostic laparoscopy in the management of trauma patients: A preliminary assessment." J Trauma 1993, 34:506–515.

31. Kuster GGR, Kline LE, Garzo G: "Diaphragmatic hernia through the foramen of Morgagni: Laparoscopic repair case report." J Laparoendosc Surg 1992, 2:93–95.

32. Yamashita YY, Bekki F, Kakegawa T, et al.: "Two laparoscopic techniques for resection of leiomyoma in the stomach." Surg Laparosc Endosc 1995, 5:38–42.

33. Pendurthi TK, DeMaria EJ, Kellum JM: "Laparoscopic bilateral inguinal hernia repair under local anesthesis." Surg Endosc 1995, 9:197–199.

34. Gazayerli M: "The Gazayerli endoscopic retractor model 1." Surg Laparosc Endosc 1991, 1:98–100.

35. Banting S, Shimi S, Velpen GV, et al.: "Abdominal wall lift: Low-pressure pneumoperitoneum laparoscopic surgery." Surg Endosc 1993, 7:57–59.

36. Inoue H, Muraoka Y, Takeshitak K, et al.: "Low-pressure pneumoperitoneum using newly devised flexible abdominal wall retractor." Surg Endosc 1993, 7:133 (Abstract).

37. Go HG, Takeda M, Imai T, et al.: "Laparoscopic adrenalectomy for Cushing's syndrome: Comparison with primary aldosteronism." Surgery 1995, 117:11–17.

5

ALTERNATIVES TO CO$_2$ PNEUMOPERITONEUM

Brian C. Organ, M.D.
Sunil K. Walia, M.D.

I. INTRODUCTION

The creation of pneumoperitoneum is a complex physiological process. Normal homeostasis is affected by increasing intraabdominal pressure and the induction of both physiological and pharmacological changes caused by diffusion of a specific gaseous agent across the peritoneal membrane. These changes are well tolerated by young and healthy patients, but elderly patients with significant cardiopulmonary comorbidity may be at an increased risk for perioperative complications. The ideal gas for pneumoperitoneum should be chemically, physiologically, and pharmacologically inert; inexpensive and readily available; and highly water soluble so that if an air embolism should occur it would rapidly dissolve in the blood stream. It should not support combustion. Carbon dioxide (CO$_2$), currently the most commonly used gas for pneumoperitoneum, possesses some of the above qualities but is associated

Abdominal Access in Open and Laparoscopic Surgery
Edited by Edmund K. M. Tsoi and Claude H. Organ, Jr.
ISBN 0-471-13352-3 Copyright © 1996 by Wiley-Liss, Inc.

with increased $PaCO_2$, end tidal CO_2 ($ETCO_2$), and decreased pH, and may cause cardiac arrhythmias and local pain.[1-4] Because of the negative effects of CO_2 there has been an increased interest in finding an alternative insufflating agent. In this chapter we will discuss our clinical experience with nitrous oxide, helium, and argon, and their use as possible alternatives to carboperitoneum. We will also review their physiological and pharmacological properties along with the advantages and disadvantages encountered with their use. Another attractive option, not reviewed in this chapter, is the use in laparoscopic surgery of mechanical devices for lifting the abdominal wall. This option is discussed at length elsewhere in the text (Chapters 7–10).

II. NITROUS OXIDE

Joseph Priestley first prepared nitrous oxide (dinitromonoxide, N_2O) in 1772. Its anesthetic properties were first demonstrated by Sir Humphrey Davy in 1800. Commercially, N_2O is produced by heating ammonium nitrate to between 245°C and 270°C.

$$NH_4NO_3 \xrightarrow{\text{Heat (245–270ºC)}} N_2O + 2H_2O$$

The process involved in drying and purifying the gas may vary from one manufacturing company to another.

Nitrous oxide is a nonirritating, sweet-smelling, and colorless gas that can be used for anesthesia. The molecular weight is 44.01 and specific gravity is 1.527 (air $\leq$ 1). It is readily compressible under 50 atmospheres of pressure at 28°C to a clear and colorless fluid with a boiling point of 89°C. It is stable in the presence of sodalime. The oil:water solubility ratio is 3:2. The blood-gas solubility coefficient is 0.47. Thus N_2O has relatively low solubility in blood (68% that of CO_2).[5] N_2O is not absorbed from the peritoneal surface quite as rapidly as CO_2 but the absorption is rapid enough so that prolonged postoperative distension usually does not occur. N_2O does not combine with hemoglobin and is carried into the blood in physical solutions only. It is excreted unchanged through the lungs except for a small fraction that escapes through the skin due to the rapid diffusion of the gas.[5]

In a recently conducted study from the University of Amsterdam, the cardiorespiratory effects of N_2O pneumoperitoneum were evaluated.[3] These changes were independent of the effect of increased intraperitoneal pressure caused by the insufflation of the gas. N_2O pneumoperitoneum caused no significant change in heart rate (HR) during insufflation phase but HR decreased during desufflation ($p < 0.05$). The mean arterial pressure (MAP) decreased from 77 ± 8 to 66 ± 15 during insufflation and increased after desufflation from 63 ± 15 to 78 ± 13. The cardiac index (CI) decreased from 3.0 ± 0.5 to 2.6 ± 0.5 $L/min/m^2$ during insufflation. This was significant when compared to CO_2 groups in the same study ($p < 0.05$). Cardiac index increased after desufflation but remained below the baseline value. Central venous pressure (CVP) increased from 5 ± 4 to 11 ± 3 and after desufflation remained high in patients in the supine position. There was no significant change in systemic vascular resistance due to N_2O pneumoperitoneum. N_2O depresses myocardial contractivity in vitro but increases the responsiveness of vascular smooth muscles to epinephrine produced by sympathetic stimulation.[5] This sympathetic stimulation is less marked with N_2O insufflation than with CO_2 pneumoperitoneum, most likely because of N_2O's analgesic effect. In patients with compromised ventricular function, N_2O may cause significant myocardial depression. The venous oxygen tension (pVO_2) and venous oxygen saturation (sVO_2) both decreased from 46 ± 6 to 35 ± 6 mm Hg and 80 ± 5 to 67 ± 11, respectively, during the insufflation phase. While both pVO_2 increased after desufflation, the sVO_2 levels remained low as compared with preinsufflation levels. Venous CO_2 tension ($pVCO_2$) and end tidal CO_2 ($ETCO_2$) were both decreased during insufflation with N_2O. After desufflation $pETCO_2$ increased but was significantly lower than that of the CO_2 group ($p < 0.05$) in the study.

In another study, N_2O produced no significant changes in either arterial $PaCO_2$ or pH.[6] Other pharmacological effects of N_2O include mild increase in cerebral blood flow and intracranial pressure. Studies on effects of N_2O on gastrointestinal motility in humans are not available. In animal models there is no marked effect in the absence of hypoxia. There is little effect on neuromuscular function in man. Skeletal muscle relaxation is not seen with N_2O. However, prolonged exposure to N_2O can depress bone marrow and chronic exposure is associated with peripheral neuropathy. There is some evidence that N_2O inhibits polymorphonuclear-neutrophil (PMN) migration and phagocytosis.[5] When N_2O is excreted from the lungs, its outward diffusion lowers the alveolar partial pressure of oxygen by about 10%. This dilutional hypoxia can be avoided by administering supplementary oxygen.

In the 1970s and 1980s, N_2O was commonly used by gynecologists and

gastroenterologists for creating pneumoperitoneum.[7–10] Its use fell into disre-
pute after reports of two cases where explosions occurred with its use. Theoretically there is always a risk of combustion from colonic gases. N_2O itself is
not flammable but it does not suppress combustion. Hydrogen and methane
are two combustible gases that are produced in the colon; hydrogen can also
be produced in as a result of bacterial overgrowth in the small bowel (for example, with an ileostomy loop or an obstructive bowel). For combustion to occur in a N_2O environment, hydrogen or methane must occupy 5.5% of the gas
volume.[11] In a recently published study from Emory University, Hunter and
his colleagues measured the concentration of combustible gases in the peritoneal cavity during several gastrointestinal laparoscopic procedures (no open
large-bowel procedures).[4] No methane was found but hydrogen was detected
in very low concentrations of 0.016–0.075% in four cases out of twenty. This
was 70 times lower than the minimum concentration necessary for combustion. In three liters of N_2O (the volume usually used to create pneumoperitoneum), at least 125 ml of 100% hydrogen or methane would be needed to
reach minimal combustible levels. Whereas the volume of all gas in the small
intestinal tract is approximately 100 ml, the volume in the colon is somewhat
higher.[12] Some gas is absorbed through the mucosa (400–1000 ml/day) and
passed as flatus. Thirty to 90% of intestinal gas is nitrogen. Furthermore, fast-
ing and bowel preparation with nonfermentable substances such as polyethylene glycol) reduces the volume of hydrogen and methane to negligible levels.
Thus it is clear that combustion could only occur as a result of burn into an un-
prepped bowel and it is unlikely that pneumoperitoneum gas would make
any difference.[4] The safe use of N_2O is further supported by the fact that over
1500 tubal ligations are performed yearly under local anesthesia with N_2O
pneumoperitoneum at Grady Memorial Hospital in Atlanta, a major teaching
facility of Emory University. There have been no instances of combustion despite the use of high-wattage, spark-inducing, bipolar electrosurgery.

   The advantages of N_2O as an agent for pneumoperitoneum are that it is
inexpensive and readily available, and that it is rapidly absorbed and eliminated from the system. Due to its analgesic effect, it causes less local pain than
CO_2 pneumoperitoneum.[2] It has minimal hemodynamic side effects as compared to CO_2 and it causes neither elevation of $PaCO_2$ nor acidosis. It may be
the ideal agent in patients with compromised cardiopulmonary function and
metabolic acidosis as well as in operations performed with local anesthesia
and intravenous sedation. N_2O insufflation may also be beneficial for pro-

longed cases, extraperitoneal dissections, and pregnant patients in whom fetal acidosis is an additional concern.[4]

The disadvantage of N_2O insufflation is its presumed inability to suppress combustion. There is always a risk of combustion in cases where the large bowel is opened. It is probably safe when used for upper gastrointestinal tract (esophagus or stomach) procedures. One might consider using CO_2 for the initial pneumoperitoneum then N_2O for the remainder of the case. Further studies will be needed to reassure surgeons regarding the safe use of N_2O.

III. HELIUM

Helium was identified in 1895 as an emanation from radioactive ore (alpha rays). In 1905, it was found in oil and gas wells in Louisiana. There is no other commercial source of the gas. Helium is marketed in compressed form in steel cylinders containing more than 95% helium, the rest being nitrogen. It is also available also in various mixtures with oxygen.[13]

Helium is a chemically and physiologically inert gas that owes its pharmacological action exclusively to its physical properties. Its molecular weight is 4.00 and its specific gravity is 0.14. The important physical properties of helium are its low density, low aqueous solubility, high thermal conductivity, and high acoustic velocity. Helium does not support combustion. It actually suppresses inflammability, though is not widely used for this purpose.[13] Dissolved helium is rapidly and totally excreted from pulmonary arterial blood into the alveoli with essentially none returned in systematic arterial blood.[13]

Apart from the general changes associated with increased intraperitoneal pressure on pulmonary function, helium insufflation does not affect $PaCO_2$ or $ETCO_2$ as does CO_2 pneumoperitoneum and causes minimal decrease in pH (during the first 45 minutes) and bicarbonate concentration. Insufflation with helium may result in increased ventilation requirements. However, one study reported that peak airway pressure increased 7 cm H_2O and there was a significant rise in alveolar-arterial oxygen gradient ($PaO_2 - PaO_2$) of 0.2 kPa.[15] The likely mechanism for this effect is that splinting of the diaphragm by the increased intraabdominal pressure caused collapse of the basal airway, which altered the ventilation and perfusion distribution, resulting in increased right–left shift and dead space.[14,15] Helium insufflation has been observed to increase the pulse rate as well as both systolic and diastolic blood pressure. These changes were independent of the insufflative agent and were probably caused by stress induced by operation.[16] Helium pneumoperitoneum does not effect cardiac output and has no antiarrhythmic effect in experimental coronary occlusion. This latter phenomenon is as yet unexplained.

Clinical experience with helium pneumoperitoneum is limited to two studies.[14,16] Results of initial reports using animals advocated helium.[17] Other therapeutic uses of helium are based on its physical properties. Its low solubility makes it useful in deep-sea diving and in prevention of decompression sickness. Helium's insolubility in body tissue is useful in pulmonary function tests where one does not wish the inspired gas to be taken up from the lung (functional residual capacity, closing volume). Its physical property of low airflow resistance is used in patients with narrowed airways.[17] The energy required to move gases in an area of respiratory obstruction with turbulent flow is inversely related to the density of the gases. As helium is so much lighter than nitrogen, a helium–oxygen mixture can be breathed with less effort than can either air or oxygen.

Helium does not produce respiratory acidosis and may be a suitable alternative for patients with severe cardiorespiratory disease undergoing laparoscopic procedures, in whom CO_2 insufflation results in excessive hypercarbia and acidosis. Also, helium insufflation does not result in significant changes in ventilation requirements. Because it is not flammable and does not support combustion it is preferable to N_2O, which theoretically supports combustion. Helium's only limitation in laparoscopic use is that it is not very water-soluble. Hence, accidental insufflation into the abdominal wall can cause surgical emphysema.[14] In addition, it is likely that helium has a lower safety margin than carbon dioxide in the event of gas embolism.[19]

IV. ARGON

In 1894 Sir William Ramsey separated a heavier element from atmospheric nitrogen. By studying this element's emission spectrum he recognized a new element and called it "argon" from the Greek for "idle" or "lazy." Argon constitutes approximately 1% of the Earth's atmosphere, from which it is commercially obtained by fractionation from liquid air for use in electric lamps, fluorescent display signs, electronic valves and as an inert gas shield in arc-welding. Argon is a member of the noble gases. It is colorless, odorless, noncombustible, and inexpensive. It is chemically nonreactive and therefore inert. Argon has an extremely low solubility in blood: 0.0305 ml gas/ml blood.

Argon has been used with increasing frequency during minimally invasive surgery in the argon-beam coagulator. Activating the coagulator effectively creates an argon pneumoperitoneum, necessitating the frequent decompression of the abdomen to release accumulated CO_2 and argon. Its ready availability in the operative suite has led to its proposed use as an insufflating agent.[20]

Only one experimental study currently exists in the literature that evaluates argon as an alternative gas for pneumoperitoneum. Eisenhauer and his colleagues at the University of California, Davis, used argon in adult pigs.[20] Using the same protocol and personnel, they collected data in their lab and compared the hemodynamic changes of argon versus N_2 and CO_2 pneumoperitoneum. They report that argon pneumoperitoneum did not affect acid–base balance or CO_2 homeostasis and therefore would make a good alternative insufflating agent to avoid the severe hypercarbia and acidemia that accompany CO_2 insufflation.[20] When compared to a nonpneumoperitoneum baseline, Eisenhauer and his associates found argon pneumoperitoneum increased inferior vena caval (IVC) pressure and systemic vascular resistance (SVR) while decreasing the cardiac index (CI) and the stroke-volume index (SVI). The rise in IVC is attributed to the direct mechanical effect of increased intraabdominal pressure secondary to pneumoperitoneum. Conversely, the decrease in CI and SVI were attributed to "argon pneumoperitoneum." The authors postulated that the decrease in SVI and CI did not occur during nitrogen pneumoperitoneum, which indicated that elevated intraabdominal pressure created by pneumoperitoneum was not the etiology. Additionally, right-atrial pressure and pulmonary-wedge pressure were not changed. This suggests that the decreased venous return did play a role in the diminished SVI and CI.[20] The increased SVR appears to have been the primary cardiovascular effect of argon pneumoperitoneum.

Andrus, in his invited commentary to the report made by Eisenhauer and his colleagues, suggests that because they did not use concurrent-control pneumoperitoneum of CO_2, nitrogen, or helium, they cannot eliminate abdominal pressure as the independent factor causing the cardiovascular changes.[21]

Motew and his colleagues performed laparoscopy at variable intraabdominal pressures in healthy anesthetized humans. At pressures up to 20 mm Hg, no changes in central venous pressure or cardiac output were noted despite moderate increases in total peripheral vascular resistance. However, as abdominal pressure exceeded 30 mm Hg, central venous pressure and cardiac output failed.[22]

The authors recommend that because these potential cardiac effects are not fully understood and may compromise patients whose cardiac status is already compromised, greater scrutiny of argon is needed before accepting it as a viable alternative to CO_2 pneumoperitoneum.[20]

V. CONCLUSION

The establishment and maintenance of pneumoperitoneum are the foundation of laparoscopic procedures. Carbon dioxide remains the gas most commonly used because it is inexpensive, readily available, readily absorbed, and rapidly eliminated. It also suppresses combustion. Disadvantages of CO_2 as an insufflation agent include potentially dangerous hypercarbia, respiratory acidosis, cardiac arrhythmias, and greater peritoneal irritation. This chapter reviewed the available data on alternative gases that may ultimately replace CO_2. For laparoscopic procedures of increasing complexity and longer duration to have applicability in older patients or those with concomitant cardiopulmonary disease, continued emphasis on discovering a safe, effective, and physiologically benign intraabdominal exposure is a necessity.

REFERENCES

1. Safran DB, Orlando R: "Physiological effects of pneumoperitoneum." Am J Surg 1994, 167:281–286.

2. Callery MP, Soper NJ: "Physiology of the pneumoperitoneum." Baillieres Clinical Gastroenterology 1993, Dec.(4):757–777.

3. Pademaker BMP, Odoom J, Dewit LT, et al.: "Haemodynamic effects of pneumoperitoneum for laparoscopic surgery: A comparison of CO_2 with N_2O insufflation." Eur J Anaesthesiol 1994, 11:301–306.

4. Hunter JG, Staheli J, Oddsdottir M, et al.: "Nitrous oxide pneumoperitoneum revisited." Surg Endosc 1995, 9:501–504.

5. Price HL: "General Anesthetics." In The Pharmacologic Basis of Therapeutics. Goodman LS, Gilman A (eds.). 5th ed. New York: Macmillan, 1975, 81–83.

6. El-Minawi MF, Wahbi O, El-Bagousi IS, et al.: "Physiologic changes during CO_2 and N_2O pneumoperitoneum in diagnostic laparoscopy." J Reprod Med 1981, 26:338–346.

7. Minoli G, Terruzzi V, Tadeo G: "Laparoscopy: The question of the proper gas." Gastrointest Endosc 1983, 29(4):325.

8. Robinson JS, Thompson JM, Wood AW: "Laparoscopy explosion hazards with nitrous oxide." Br Med J 1975, 2:765.

9. Scott DB: "Cardiac arrhythmia during laparoscopy." Br Med J 1972, 2:49–50.

10. Scott DB, Julian DG: "Observation on cardiac arrhythmia during laparoscopy. Br Med J 1972, 1:411–413.

11. Lewis B, vonElbe G: Combustion, Flames and Explosion of Gases, 3d ed. Orlando, FL: Academic Press, 1987, 706–709.

12. Schrock T: "Large Intestine." In Current Surgical Diagnosis and Treatment. Way L (ed.). 8th ed. New York: Appelton and Lange, 1988, 588.

13. Smith TC, Gross JB, Wellman H: "The Therapeutic Gases." In The Pharmacologic Basis of Therapeutics. Goodman LS, Gilman A (eds.). 5th ed. New York: Macmillan, 1975, 897–898.

14. McMahon AJ, Baxter JN, O'Dwyer PJ, et al.: "Helium pneumoperitoneum for laparoscopic cholecystectomy: Ventilatory and blood gas changes." Br J Surg 1994, 81:1033–1036.

15. Brown DR, Fishburne JI, Robertson VO, et al.: "Ventilatory and blood gas changes during laparoscopy with local anesthesia." Am J Obstet Gynecol 1976, 124:741–745.

16. Bongard FS, Pianim NA, Leighton TA, et al.: "Helium insufflation for laparoscopic operation." Surg Gynecol Obstet 1993, 177:140–146.

17. Leighton TA, Bongard FS, Liu ST, et al.: "Comparative cardiopulmonary effects of helium and carbon dioxide pneumoperitoneum." Surg Forum 1991, 62:485–487.

18. Fleming MD, Weight JA, Brewer V, et al.: "Effect of helium and oxygen on airflow in a narrowed airway." Arch Surg 1992, 127:956–959.

19. Graff TD, Arbegast NR, Phillips OC, et al.: "Gas embolism: A comparative study of air and carbon dioxide as embolic agents in the systemic venous system." Am J Obstet Gynecol 1959, 78:259–265.

20. Eisenhauer DM, Saunders CJ, Ho HS, et al.: "Hemodynamic effects of argon pneumoperitoneum." Surg Endosc 1994, 8:315–321.

21. Andrus CH: "Invited commentary: Hemodynamic effects of argon pneumoperitoneum." Surg Endosc 1994, 8:322–323.

22. Motew M, Ivankovich AD, Bieniarz J, et al.: "Cardiovascular effects and acid-base and blood gas changes during laparoscopy." Am J Obstet Gynecol 1973, 115:1002–1012.

6

COMPLICATIONS OF CO$_2$ PNEUMOPERITONEUM

Diana M. Vogt, M.D.*
Lawrence J. Goldstein, M.D.†
Elsa R. Hirvela, M.D‡

I. INTRODUCTION

Minimally invasive surgery has enjoyed growing popularity since laparoscopic cholecystectomy was first introduced by Mouret in 1987. However, along with initial enthusiasm for this growing field, have come reports of complications unique to this new technology. Early reports of laparoscopic complications were published in the gynecological literature. In these reviews, laparoscopy was almost exclusively performed in young healthy women, and the procedures were minor or diagnostic in nature. Expanding application of minimally invasive surgery to more advanced procedures in older and less

*Section II.
†Section III.
‡Section IV.

Abdominal Access in Open and Laparoscopic Surgery
Edited by Edmund K. M. Tsoi and Claude H. Organ, Jr.
ISBN 0-471-13352-3 Copyright © 1996 by Wiley-Liss, Inc.

healthy general-surgery patients has resulted in additional complications that fall outside the realm of conventional open surgery.[1] An awareness of potential pitfalls of advanced laparoscopic surgical techniques will facilitate recognition and avoidance of these complications. This chapter will focus on the various complications related to laparoscopic surgery. In addition, methods to avoid these potential problems will be suggested.

II. VISCERAL AND ABDOMINAL-WALL COMPLICATIONS

The ability to perform laparoscopic surgery is predicated on the need for a working space in the abdomen in order to visualize intraabdominal structures and to use instruments to perform the operation. The most common means of creating this space is by insufflating gas into the peritoneal cavity. Placement of a Veress needle is often the method used to initially instill gas into the peritoneum. As mentioned in Chapter 3, CO_2 is the most commonly used gas because it is inexpensive, readily available, does not support combustion, and has a high diffusion coefficient so that it is rapidly absorbed across the peritoneum and then excreted via the lungs.[1] After CO_2 insufflation, laparoscopic ports through which instruments can be inserted are placed into the abdominal space. At any point in the creation of the peritoneal space or placement of the ports, injury to the abdominal wall or visceral structures can occur. In addition, CO_2 can be insufflated into spaces other than the peritoneum, creating additional complications. Because of the lack of three-dimensional viewing with the laparoscope, injuries due to past-pointing with sharp instruments or cautery are encountered more frequently in laparoscopic procedures than in conventional surgery. Finally, hernias can develop through the fascial defects at the port sites, with the potential problem of incarceration.

Incidence

Complications secondary to pneumoperitoneum creation via the Veress needle, CO_2 insufflation, and trocar placement occur in 0.1–0.5% of cases.[2] The most common Veress-needle problems involve misinsufflation of CO_2 and injury to the vessels, bowel, and bladder. Incisional hernias have been reported to occur in 0.1% of laparoscopic cases, with the umbilical port being the most common site.[3] The incidence of cautery injuries in laparoscopic surgery is unknown, but is likely more common than in open procedures.

Mechanism, Recognition, and Management

The creation of the pneumoperitoneum and the placement of the initial trocar into the abdomen result in more morbidity than the placement of the secondary trocars, which are introduced under direct visualization after the camera has been inserted. Injuries occur because the Veress needle and the initial trocar are placed without visual guidance. Current instruments include numerous safety features in an attempt to avert these injuries to various organs (for instance, the bowel, bladder, stomach, and solid organs).[7–9] Carbon dioxide insufflation into spaces other than the peritoneum may result in subcutaneous emphysema, air in visceral organs, or air embolism.[2] The inability to create a pneumoperitoneum is a common reason for converting from a laparoscopic to an open procedure.[6]

Diagnosis of bowel, bladder, or stomach injury can be made soon after the Veress needle is placed by immediately aspirating the needle with a syringe. If intestinal contents are seen in the syringe, the diagnosis of full-thickness bowel injury is made.[6] The Veress needle should be removed and an open technique used to achieve pneumoperitoneum. The camera should then be placed and the abdomen endoscopically surveyed to assess the extent of injury. The treatment will depend on the degree of injury. Full-thickness perforations, demonstrated by intestinal contents freely spilling into the abdomen, require repair. If the operating surgeon is facile in endoscopic suturing techniques, repair of bowel lacerations can occasionally be performed laparoscopically.[6] Most often, however, open repair is necessary.[9] If intestinal contents are aspirated but no spillage of enteric contents are seen when the abdomen is inspected, the injury may have been only partial—thickness and may seal on its own, in which case further treatment is unnecessary. If the injured bowel is adherent to the abdominal wall adjacent to the umbilical port, the injury can be inspected by placing the second port, inserting the camera in this port, and then surveying the damage from this viewpoint.

Bladder perforations are diagnosed when urine is aspirated through the Veress needle or when air or blood is seen in the Foley catheter drainage bag. These injuries usually occur because of the failure to decompress the bladder prior to inserting the needle. Additionally, patients who have had previous pelvic surgery may have an abnormally positioned bladder. Veress needle bladder perforations, because of their small size, usually do not need to be repaired and may be managed by postoperative catheter drainage.[9] Trocar injuries to the bowel and bladder are more extensive than those caused by the Veress needle and almost always require conversion to an open procedure for repair.[9]

Incorrect placement of the Veress needle may also result in misinsufflation of CO$_2$. When CO$_2$ is insufflated anterior to the rectus sheath, subcutaneous emphysema results. Subcutaneous emphysema also occurs when the skin incision is too large and air leaks around the port. Diagnosis is established when the abdomen is seen to distend asymmetrically and crepitation is palpated.[9,10] Subcutaneous emphysema in and of itself is not usually clinically significant, as CO$_2$ is rapidly absorbed. However, massive subcutaneous emphysema leading to hypercarbia requiring prolonged intubation has been reported.[11] Additionally, subcutaneous air can dissect upward through a diaphragmatic defect resulting in pneumothorax or pneumomediastinum.[9] Carbon dioxide insufflation into the space between the fascia and peritoneum results in properitoneal emphysema. This is usually diagnosed when the camera is placed and the peritoneum is found to still be intact and properitoneal fat is seen. Carbon dioxide should be evacuated from the properitoneal space and an open technique for trocar placement should be employed.[6] Insufflation of carbon dioxide into the mesentery or retroperitoneum can result in pneumomediastinum, pneumopericardium, or pneumothorax.[2]

Carbon dioxide embolism, one of the most devastating potential complications, is fortunately also one of the most rare complications of gas misinsufflation (see the Section IV, below).

Electrocautery injuries to the bowel, bladder, and blood vessels have been reported in laparoscopic surgery.[8,11] The most common reason for thermal injury is failure to ground the patient adequately.[2] If diagnosed intraoperatively, the injury can be treated conservatively with bowel rest and intravenous antibiotics.[6] Because of the difficulty of visualization in laparoscopic surgery, the injuries may not be immediately recognized resulting in morbidity and mortality.[2,6] Many patients undergoing laparoscopic surgery are discharged home soon after their procedures. However symptoms of thermal injury may not occur until 3–7 days postoperatively. Patients who present with fever, nausea, abdominal pain, and leukocytosis should initially be treated with antibiotics. If there is not an immediate response or if peritonitis develops, exploration is mandatory. Thermal damage may be more extensive than the superficial injury may appear; so resection of all potentially injured tissue should be done. The abdomen should be drained and IV antibiotics continued for 7–10 days.[6]

The use of electrocautery in the presence of CO_2 can create carbon monoxide (CO).[12] Increased levels of intraperitoneal CO can lead to increased systemic CO and increased blood carboxyhemoglobin levels. The significance, if any, of increased intraperitoneal CO is not yet known.[12]

Despite the small size of the incisions used to place ports, herniation through fascial defects at the port sites has been reported postoperatively.[2] Incarcerated hernias and Richter's hernias have both been described in the literature.[13–15] Umbilical port site herniation is most commonly reported. The small, rigid, fascial defect at this site makes the development of Richter's hernias possible. Treatment is no different from that of any incisional hernia.

Prevention

Many of the complications presented are due to technical errors and can be prevented by adhering to some simple but effective techniques. There are a number of maneuvers that should be used routinely to prevent abdominal organ injury. A nasogastric tube should always be placed to decompress the stomach before inserting any instruments into the abdomen.[6] Many surgeons also advocate routine urinary catheter placement prior to creating the pneumoperitoneum, although the bladder can be decompressed by having the patient void just before entering the operating room.[2] The patient should be placed in the Trendelenburg position so that the stomach and colon will fall away from the umbilical area. Additionally, lifting the abdominal wall can reduce the incidence of visceral injury by providing counter traction during instrument insertion and by increasing the distance between the instrument and the abdominal and retroperitoneal structures.[9] Trocars should never be inserted until adequate pneumoperitoneum, as evidenced by intraabdominal pressures of at least 12 mm Hg, has been attained. When patients have had prior abdominal operations, the possibility of adhesions to the anterior abdominal wall increases the risk of bowel or bladder injury.[6] In these situations, serious consideration should be given to using an open technique in which a blunt-tipped Hasson cannula is placed into the peritoneal cavity under direct visualization and CO_2 is then insufflated.[16]

Prevention of CO_2 misinsufflation requires verifying correct Veress nee-

dle placement prior to initiating gas flow. After placing the Veress needle, a syringe should be attached and aspirated. If air is aspirated, the saline drop test
should then be performed.[6] This test consists of placing saline in the hub of the
needle and lifting the anterior abdominal wall. The negative intraabdominal
pressure should cause the saline to drop into the abdomen if the needle is correctly positioned. As insufflation is initiated, the pressure monitor should be
watched closely. At low gas flows, the intraabdominal pressures should remain low, usually less than 5 mm Hg, and should vary with respiration. If the
initial pressure is higher than this or if the pressure increases quickly at low
flow, the needle should be assumed to be incorrectly placed and should be
redirected. Finally, during insufflation, the abdomen itself should be observed
for symmetrical distension and loss of hepatic dullness to percussion. If at any
point in this sequence of events there is difficulty, the surgeon should maintain
a low threshold for switching to the previously described open technique in
which a blunt-tipped catheter is placed in the abdomen under direct visualization after an periumbilical cutdown incision has been made.

The obese patient represents a particular challenge, since routine laparoscopic instruments may not be long enough to get through the thick layer of
tissue between the skin and the peritoneum. Extra-long Veress needles are
available and may be used in this situation. However, if there is any difficulty
in placing the Veress needle or confirming its correct position, an open approach should be used.

Electrocautery injuries can be prevented first and foremost by correctly
grounding the patient.[2] Additionally, the cautery should be applied carefully
for the minimal amount of time needed to achieve results. The activated
cautery tip should not be moved from one place to another in a closed space,
and should only be activated when the tip is directly on the tissue to be cauterized; past-pointing should be avoided. Finally, The instruments should always
be checked to assure that they are adequately insulated. This is particularly
important when reusable instruments with cautery attachments are used. Visual inspection of the entire instrument should be performed prior to using any
instrument that has been used and sterilized repeatedly in order to ensure that
the insulation is intact.

To prevent the entirely avoidable incidence of postoperative trocar-site
herniation, there are a number of techniques that should be routinely employed. When possible, small trocars should be used. Air should be completely

evacuated prior to removing the trocars so that the added intraperitoneal pressure does not cause omentum or viscera to prolapse through the trocar sites. Trocars should be removed under direct visualization whenever possible to assure that herniation has not occurred.[2] The fascia of 10 mm trocar insertion sites should be closed when technically feasible.[14] The anterior sheath of fascial incisions should always be closed in situations when fascial enlargement has been necessary in order to remove organs.[9] If the open technique is used to gain entry into the abdomen, fascial sutures should be placed prior to inserting the Hasson cannula. This will facilitate closing the fascia at the conclusion of the procedure.

III. VASCULAR COMPLICATIONS OF MINIMALLY INVASIVE SURGERY

Incidence

The exact incidence of vascular injury in minimally invasive surgery is not known, but it is low. Most injuries occur during the insertion of the pneumoperitoneum needle or trocar, but they can occur during the course of the procedure as well.[28] Injury can befall the great abdominal and pelvic vessels, which include the aorta, inferior vena cava, iliac arteries, and veins,[17] as well as mesenteric and omental vessels and the inferior epigastric artery. One series, from Loffer and Pent, as well as Kuzel and Edingen[3] reported 6.4 incidents of vascular injury for every thousand cases, but most of these injuries involved superficial vessels. Baadsgaard[18] and Caprini[19] uncovered only 19 injuries in 30,000 laparoscopies, most of which involved the aorta (8), iliac artery (7), and, less commonly, the common iliac vein, the superior mesenteric artery, a jejunal artery branch, or an abdominal-wall bleeder (one each). In this study, the Veress needle was responsible for as many injuries as the subumbilical trocar (six cases each), but the potential severity of the injury is much higher for the subumbilical trocar. Other studies[17] have revealed that the trocar was the most common cause of the vascular injury. The incidence of anterior abdominal wall hemorrhage is 2.5 to 6 cases per 1,000 laparoscopies, according to Loffer and Pent,[3] Lieberman,[4] and Chamberlain.[5] McDonald and Rich[20] reported that physicians who have performed fewer than 100 laparoscopic procedures have about four times more vascular complications as those with a greater experience (14.7 per thousand procedures versus 3.8 per thousand procedures).

Mechanism

Inexperienced, unskilled, or careless personnel probably account for the majority of injuries,[3,10,22] but even seasoned surgeons have these complications, especially in unusual circumstances. When a trocar becomes dull or the physician fails to rotate the trocar, the insertion requires more pressure and may lead to a loss of control and inadvertent laceration of intraabdominal and retroperitoneal structures. In addition, the problems noted above (Section I) pertain. Any forceful, uncontrolled thrust during insertion is an obvious risk factor for vascular injury, as is failure to use the appropriate landmarks for needle or trocar insertion.

Special Considerations

Slender patients are at increased risk for vascular injury because there may be only a half inch separating their skin from the abdominal aorta. Patients with portal hypertension have a patent umbilical vein 34% of the time,[24] and, therefore, should a needle pierce this hypertensive venous structure, it could have life-threatening consequences. In one French study, there was an incidence of four such occurrences out of 35,000 laparoscopies.[24] Unfortunately, because of the structure involved, it may be 30 minutes or more after completion of the laparoscopy before there is any evidence of injury.

In addition, such conditions as diastasis recti, adhesive abdomen, rich abdominal-wall collaterals from peripheral vascular disease or portal hypertension, and pronounced lumbar lordosis may put the patient at added risk.

Obese patients may require a needle insertion angle of as little as 10° from the normal[22] and are therefore predisposed to vascular injuries on that basis. In patients with previous periumbilical incisions, one must avoid the periumbilical vascular ring and make an attempt to aim the trocar towards the pelvis to stay away from these adhesions. Some authors recommend a Z technique in entering the abdominal wall after aiming the trocar subcutaneously for several centimeters prior to entering the peritoneum.[27] Patients who have had a previous vascular prosthesis, such as the thoracoiliac, femoral, or aortoiliac bypass, are at increased risk of injury, not only due to the previous operation but because of the location of the graft, and these conditions should be taken into account when minimally invasive procedures are entertained in these patients.

Anatomy

The umbilicus is traditionally thought to mark the location of the abdominal aortic bifurcation, but Penfield has pointed out that the position of the umbilicus is highly variable (especially in the obese).[22] Even when compared to a fixed landmark, the aortic bifurcation is not necessarily at the level of L4 or the iliac crest. Goss has found that the aortic bifurcation occurs within 1.25 cm of L4 in 80% of cases.[23] In 9% it lies above L4, and in 11%, below the L4–L5 cartilage (Figure 6.1).

Anatomy of the Inferior Epigastric Artery

The inferior epigastric artery arises from the external iliac artery behind the conjoint tendon over the circular fold of Douglas and enters the rectus abdominis sheath to anastomose with the superior epigastric artery (a branch of the

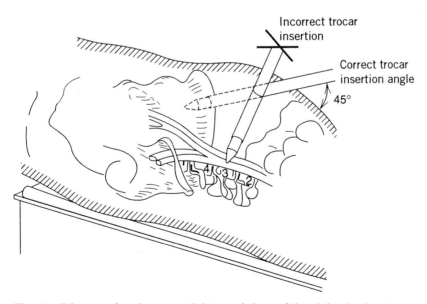

Fig. 6.1. Diagram showing potential trocar injury of the abdominal aorta.

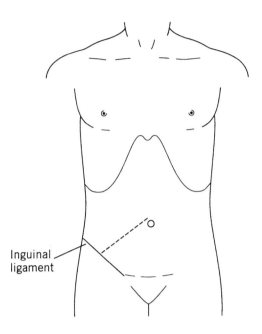

Fig. 6.2. Diagram depicting the course of the inferior epigastric artery.

internal thoracic). The inferior epigastric artery runs along a line joining the mid inguinal ligament to a point just lateral to the umbilicus (Figure 6.2). One can avoid anterior-wall hemorrhage from the inferior epigastric artery by staying at least 1 cm from the known course of the vessel, by a midline approach, or by puncturing the lateral edge of the rectus abdominis. The peritoneal needle should be placed at a 45° angle to the pelvis with the patient in the Trendelenburg position to prevent injury to the omentum and great abdominal vessels (use caution in the obese patient).

The technique of open laparoscopy championed by Penfield and originally described by Hassen[17] is said to have no risk of a major vascular injury; but even in experienced hands, albeit less often, major vascular injuries do occur. In patients with portal hypertension, caput medusae, venous murmurs, or ultrasound visualization of the umbilical vein, if a patent vein is noted, we recommend that the surgeon put the trocar a few centimeters below the umbilicus to avoid it or use open cannulation. In patients with suspected abdominal-wall adhesions, preoperative ultrasound mapping of the adhesions to guide placement of the trocar or a peritoneal needle can be helpful, or, better yet, prompt an open technique in needle placement.[20]

What to Do for a Suspected Vascular Injury

If one encounters difficulty in placing the Veress needle and any of the following signs occur, one should be suspicious of a vascular injury: blood in the hub
of the Veress needle, even a few drops, but especially if under pressure; a
marked drop in blood pressure or tachycardia; and abdominal distension noted
after the early attempts to place the needle (before insufflation).[26] If any of these
signs occur, immediate laparotomy is warranted without waiting for other evidence of intraabdominal bleeding and before the patient goes into severe shock.

If the vascular injury was not suspected after placing the peritoneal needle, or if the injury was due to the trocar and one is already in the abdomen,
one can scan the abdomen with the camera to rule out a vascular injury. When
blood is found in the peritoneal needle, it should be left in place for repeated
aspirations to help make the diagnosis.[27] In the postoperative period, if the patient is hypotensive, a major vascular injury should be considered, as it may
have been unrecognized during the procedure.[22]

Carbon dioxide insufflation (more than 150–200 cc/min.) can be responsible for gas embolization and should be treated as noted below (Section
IV).

Repairing Injured Vessels

For skin and subcutaneous bleeding, a combination of cautery and suture ligation should be utilized. For the inferior epigastric artery, ligation with perma-
nent suture material is recommended. The incision may have to be extended
for proper isolation of the epigastric artery after evacuation of the hematoma.
Bleeding of branches of the mesenteric vessels or omental artery or veins may
require a laparotomy and suture ligation, or it can be controlled with minimally invasive techniques or cautery, depending on the individual situation. If tissue has been transected either accidentally or by coagulation but inadequately
fulgurated, recoagulation or clip ligation may prevent open laparotomy. Injuries to the aorta may be amenable to lateral suture repair with or without
proximal and distal control, with or without heparin. If the surgeon feels that
the arteriotomy or venotomy can be repaired within a few minutes, one can
clamp the aorta and common iliac arteries with impunity without heparin;
however, if an extended period of time for repair is anticipated, heparinization
with 100 units/kg intravenous administration is recommended until the acti-

vated clotting (ACT) is twice normal. Small anterior arteriotomies can be repaired by placing a finger over the laceration, suturing at the apex of the arteriotomy, and closing transversely with a 3 to 5-0 proline suture. As the stitches advance, the occluding finger can be retracted to prevent bleeding. Alternately, if one is uncomfortable with that technique, the proximal aorta can be occluded either with finger pressure or aortic occlusion devices or direct aortic clamping. If back bleeding from the iliac arteries is more than can be tolerated during the repair, those can be clamped as well.

Injuries to the bifurcation may not be amenable to lateral-suture repair and may necessitate short bifurcated grafts or advancement of the bifurcation. Polytetrafluruethylene (PTFE) or dacron are equally effective in this circumstance if intraabdominal contamination has not occurred. If there is a major injury to an iliac vein or cava in a region that is difficult to get to due to the overlying iliac arteries, the iliac artery or aorta can be transected after heparin is given to allow exposure to the venous injuries underneath. It is best not to handle the iliac vein or caval injuries in the same manner as arterial injuries in that they do not tolerate cross-clamping as well due to their thin, friable nature. In order to get access to the venous injury, the overlying artery either must be mobilized or transected to allow the venous repair, and then arterial reanastomosis or repair can follow.

In cases of an arterio–venous fistula, because of its acute nature, primary closure of the individual injured vessels and placement of viable tissue between them is all that is necessary. In all instances, whenever significant intraabdominal bleeding is encountered, first apply direct pressure to stop the bleeding and then assess the injury. Then proximal and distal control, when needed, can be obtained.

Results of Repair. Recovery is the rule. However, in one series, two patients out of 15 succumbed to their injury due to complications of hypovolemic shock.[19] The actual statistics are unknown at the present time for the more complex and sicker patients undergoing minimally invasive operations.

Venous Physiology

Incidence. Deep venous thrombosis and pulmonary embolism in laparoscopic procedures for gynecologic reasons is rare. In one study, in only 0.2 in

1,000 procedures did this occur.[29] However, in one laparoscopic cholecystectomy series, two patients out of 487 developed this complication.[30] In laparoscopic cholecystectomy and in other longer operations, the incidence may be higher, similar to that in open procedures.

Pathophysiology

The intraperitoneal pressure from the CO_2 gas decreases venous return. To compound the mechanical effects of the pneumoperitoneum in decreasing venous return, the reverse Trendelenburg position produces decrements in venous return as well. General anesthesia by itself decreases lower-limb venous return and increase venous stasis, similar to 10–14 days of bed rest. Finally, hypercoagulability due to release of tissue thromboplastin at the operative site increases the number of platelets and adhesiveness, and decreased fibrolytic activity associated with operation occurs in some patients, but is no different from the hypercoagulability caused by the open technique. Common femoral venous diameter increases an average of 30% with a 12-mm Hg pneumoperitoneum.[29] Intermittent pneumatic compression can abolish much of the effects of the pneumoperitoneum and reverse Trendelenburg position.[29] Peak systolic velocity of the common femoral vein has been found to decrease from 0.24 ± 0.025 to 0.14 ± 0.011 m/sec (a 42% decrease following 12-mm Hg pneumoperitoneum). Intermittent compression stockings reverse that effect completely (to 0.27 ± 0.021 m/sec). Anesthesia alone increased the velocity to 0.30 ± 0.032 m/sec. The mean arterial pressure hardly changed.[31] Finally, Moneta reported a decreased velocity secondary to the reverse Trendelenburg position.[32]

Prevention

We recommend intermittent pneumatic compression stockings perioperatively for all patients receiving a pneumoperitoneum. Subcutaneous or intravenous heparin should be considered, depending on the patient's underlying risk factors and should be appropriate for the procedure being performed. One should also consider operating on the patient in the flat position if this is technically feasible, as the reverse Trendelenburg position detrimentally affects the venous return. Finally, treat the patient's underlying condition as you would in open procedures.

IV. PULMONARY AND HEMODYNAMIC COMPLICATIONS

Incidence

The incidence of cardiopulmonary complications in the patient population historically undergoing laparoscopy—healthy young women—was exceedingly rare. Although there were isolated reports of serious complications such as arrhythmia and gas embolus, the literature antedating the laparoscopic revolution in general surgery is reassuringly devoid of any common cardiac or pulmonary side effects of laparoscopic operations.

For a variety of reasons, this historic data cannot be freely extrapolated to the realm of contemporary laparoscopy in the general surgical population. Indications for minimally invasive surgery have expanded, and more complex procedures are now undertaken laparoscopically. High-risk patients, including the acute trauma patient, the elderly, and the patient unable to tolerate an open procedure, are now managed laparoscopically. Because of their complexity, procedures are longer and patients are frequently subject to pneumoperitoneum for periods far in excess of the time needed for gynecologic diagnosis or therapy.

Thus, the true incidence of cardiopulmonary complications that arise as the result of pneumoperitoneum is as yet unknown. What is known, from the results of early case reports, small clinical trials, and animal experimentation, is that such complications will be more prevalent than in the historic group, and that risk factors for such complications can be identified.

The contemporary laparoscopic surgeon should have a working knowledge of the cardiopulmonary side effects of CO₂ pneumoperitoneum, and should be able to determine whether his or her patients carry an increased risk for their occurrence. The surgeon should be able to identify cardiopulmonary side effects when they occur, and be capable of instituting the appropriate corrective measures.

Gas Embolus

Gas embolus during laparoscopy has been reported to occur with a frequency of 0.09% to 0.002%.[29] The emboli usually occur on the venous side of the circulation, as gas under the positive pressure of pneumoperitoneum is forced into the low-pressure venous system. Such a mechanism dictates that the emboli are usually small, except in incidences of direct venopuncture by the Veress needle or large venous injuries. Arterial emboli are much rarer, occurring as the result of direct arterial insufflation of CO_2 following accidental arterial puncture. Another potential arterial source is paradoxical embolus of CO_2 from the venous to the arterial side via a patent foramen ovale. Since the positive pressure of pneumoperitoneum should never exceed arterial pressure, direct transarterial embolization of CO_2 is not of concern.

Carbon dioxide embolus should be suspected in the setting of pneumoperitoneum if the patient develops sudden and profound hypotension. If the precordium is accessible for auscultation, or a transesophageal stethoscope is in place, a machinery murmur will be heard. The transesophageal stethoscope is capable of detecting small amounts of intravenous or intracardiac gas, providing an early warning of CO_2 embolus.

When CO_2 embolus occurs, the patient should be immediately placed in the left lateral decubitis position so that any CO_2 in the right heart will rise laterally in the ventricle, away from the pulmonary outflow track. Insufflation of CO_2 should be terminated. Insufflated CO_2 carbon dioxide is highly soluble in blood, so that even large amounts are rapidly reabsorbed. For this reason, if cardiac arrest occurs as the result of a CO_2 embolus, the patient should be returned to a supine position and CPR instituted. Resuscitation is often possible.

Hypercapnia

Both in experimental models and in humans undergoing laparoscopic surgery with CO_2 pneumoperitoneum, increases in arterial CO_2 with corresponding decreases in pH have been detected.[1,34,35] In a porcine model, eight pigs underwent CO_2 pneumoperitoneum at 15 mm Hg for 60 minutes. Arterial CO_2 rose from a baseline of 34.5 mm Hg to a maximum of 48.6 mm Hg. pH fell from 7.47 to a minimum of 7.35.[36]

As laparoscopic procedures become more prolonged, increasing numbers of patients with significant hypercapnia, requiring termination of the pneumoperitoneum or prolonged postoperative intubation, are being reported. This has been particularly true in the high-risk pulmonary group, a patient population in whom laparoscopic surgery is preferentially selected to avoid the detrimental side effects of large abdominal incisions on postoperative pulmonary function.

Recent clinical experience makes it evident that patients who fall in an American Society of Anesthesiology (ASA) class II or class III on the basis of poor pulmonary function require particularly careful monitoring for the development of both intraoperative and postoperative hypercapnia. Even the routine use of end-tidal CO$_2$ monitoring in these patients may not provide sufficient early warning that significant acidemia is developing.

In a recent analysis of 30 patients undergoing laparoscopic cholecystectomy with a mean operating time of approximately 170 minutes, a subset of 10 ASA II and III patients demonstrated a significant rise in CO$_2$ compared to the 20 ASA I patients (46.1 versus 36.6 mm Hg) and a significant fall in pH (7.33 versus 7.4). In the high-risk group, two patients had to be converted to open cholecystectomy because of a severe, persistent acidosis. End-tidal CO$_2$ increased in both groups but was not statistically significantly different, nor did arterial pO$_2$ discriminate between those with significant hypercapnia and those without.[2] These authors note that end-tidal CO$_2$ was only slightly changed even in the face of severely deranged pH and pCO$_2$ values.

Because CO$_2$ readily diffuses through cell membranes, excess CO$_2$ that is not excreted by the lungs during operation dissolves in muscle and soft tissue, to be slowly released into the circulation postoperatively. With marginal pulmonary function, this increased demand on ventilation may exceed the patient's ability to respond unless prolonged ventilator support is supplied until tissue CO$_2$ levels return to normal.

It is evident that close monitoring of *arterial pH and CO$_2$* by frequent arterial blood-gas determinations or a continuous indwelling arterial blood-gas monitor is imperative for patients with underlying pulmonary disorders who will undergo CO$_2$ pneumoperitoneum. Identification of such high-risk patients preoperatively with the appropriate anesthesia consultation and preoperative pulmonary evaluation is of the greatest value in avoiding intraoperative and postoperative misadventures due to profound acid–base disturbances.

In the event that rising CO$_2$ is found to be causing an unacceptable fall in pH intraoperatively, minute ventilation can be increased in an effort to normalize values. This can be accomplished by increasing rate, tidal volume, or both. Increases in tidal volume are limited by accompanying increases in airway pressure. At high tidal volumes, airway pressures will increase to dangerously high levels, with an increased risk of barotrauma and increase in right-ventricular work (see below) Increases in rate must be tempered by the need to provide enough time for full exhalation, or breath stacking and autopeep can occur. Normally, expiration takes twice as long as inspiration, but in those with an underlying airways disease (such as asthma, or chronic obstructive pulmonary disease), expiration may be prolonged.

If the pH and CO_2 cannot be stabilized within a safe range, CO_2 insufflation should be discontinued and the operation should be converted to a gasless laparoscopic approach or an open procedure. Close monitoring of pH and CO_2 should be continued postoperatively in a recovery room or ICU setting.

Extubation should not be contemplated until the patient has returned to his baseline values of pH and CO_2. Even at this point, a trial of spontaneous breathing on a T-piece may be highly desirable, to insure the patient's ability to maintain adequate CO_2 homeostasis without ventilator support.

Mechanics of Ventilation

In addition to increased demands on minute ventilation, the effects of CO_2 pneumoperitoneum and patient positioning on the mechanics of breathing cannot be ignored. Pneumoperitoneum can necessitate increases in peak airway pressure to provide and adequate tidal volume. This can result in an increased risk for acute complications of barotrauma such as pneumothorax and tension pneumothorax.

If the patient needs to be placed in Trendelenberg to facilitate exposure, as is particularly the case in the lower abdomen and pelvis, additional impairment of diaphragmatic excursion may result, requiring further increments in ventilatory pressure to deliver an appropriate tidal volume.

Finally, there is a small incidence of cases in which pneumothorax or tension pneumothorax has developed as the result of direct communication of the pleural space with the peritoneal space. This is of particular concern when transdiaphragmatic pathology (such as large hiatus or diaphragmatic hernia), or penetrating trauma to the diaphragm is present.

Sudden large increases in peak airway pressure, particularly if accompanied by hypotension, should lead to the immediate suspicion of a tension pneumothorax. Carbon dioxide insufflation should be terminated and the pneumoperitoneum should be immediately released. Auscultation for the unilateral absence of breath sounds should lead to the rapid placement of a large-bore intravenous catheter in the second intercostal space on the appropriate side. Decompression should not be delayed for a chest-tube set or a chest x ray.

Once definitive treatment has been instituted, a decision should be made about the safety or necessity of proceeding.

Peak airway pressures below 40 cm of water are associated with a negligible incidence of barotrauma, so increases below this point usually require no intervention. If the patient becomes progressively more difficult to ventilate with the establishment of the pneumoperitoneum, a number of strategies can be considered.

Incomplete muscle relaxation may contribute significantly to chest-wall stiffness so that completely paralyzing the patient improves chest-and abdominal-wall compliance, resulting in lower airway pressures. Pneumoperitoneum pressures lower than the conventionally chosen 15 cm of water may permit adequate exposure without compromising the surgeon's ability to perform the procedure laparoscopically. Conversion to a gasless laparoscopic technique with an external lifting device may also be an option.

Altering the position of the patient so that abdominal contents are more dependent to the diaphragm can also help improve the mechanics of breathing. It may be acceptable to ventilate the patient more rapidly with smaller tidal volumes, thus maintaining minute ventilation while decreasing peak airway pressures. Finally, if efforts to reduce peak airway pressures with the abdomen closed fail, the operation should be converted to an open mode.

Arrhythmias

Arrhythmias occurring as the result of CO$_2$ pneumoperitoneum run the gamut from transient bradycardias to tachyarrhythmias, ventricular ectopy, and full cardiac arrest.[37,38] Distension of the peritoneal cavity to create a pneumoperitoneum may result in a vagally mediated bradycardia, which usually responds to atropine and is transient in nature. Catecholamine-induced ectopy occurs only marginally more often than in patients undergoing open procedures under general anesthesia and need not impair the progression of the operation if it can be suppressed. Scott and Julian[37] compared the incidence of arrhythmias in patients undergoing CO$_2$ pneumoperitoneum and N$_2$O pneumoperitoneum. Arrhythmias were far more common with CO$_2$. Most consisted of premature ventricular heats, although ventricular tachycardia occurred in several.

Far more difficult to treat are those arrhythmias that arise from serious acid–base disturbances as the result of undetected CO$_2$ retention. It is probably this last mechanism that is responsible for the majority of cardiac arrests occurring in the setting of laparoscopic surgery (0.03%).[38] CPR should be instituted immediately, with immediate release of pneumoperitoneum. Tension pneumothorax and CO_2 embolus should be quickly ruled out as precipitating causes. It may be worthwhile to administer bicarbonate, even in the absence of an increase in end-tidal CO_2, since significant acidosis may still be present and hyperventilation may not correct the pH as rapidly if there is underlying lung disease.

Cardiac Pump Function

Carbon dioxide pneumoperitoneum can alter every determinant of cardiac performance, including preload, afterload, and myocardial contractility. Early work on the hemodynamic consequences of pneumoperitoneum tended to focus on the mechanical aspects of impaired venous return and increased splanchnic resistance as the primary sources of impaired cardiac function.[39,40] Since pressure in the inferior vena cava is normally in the 8–12 cm of water range, compression by a pneumoperitoneum at usual insufflation pressures is possible, resulting in inhibition of venous return from the lower extremities and abdominal viscera. In reality, pneumoperitoneum has no clinically significant effect on central venous pressure and venous return in the euvolemic, supine patient.[36] Central venous pressure may fall if such patients are positioned in reverse Trendelenberg, although the hemodynamic effects are usually inconsequential.[41]

In hypovolemic patients, particularly those who may be undergoing laparoscopy for trauma, the effect of pneumoperitoneum on venous return can contribute to precipitous drops in cardiac output and blood pressure. Wolf and colleagues[42] demonstrated that animals undergoing pneumoperitoneum following even mild hemorrhage could experience significant decreases in cardiac index and mean arterial pressure, which only transiently responded to subsequent fluid resuscitation. The effect could not be explained by changes in arterial CO_2 or pH alone.

Carbon dioxide pneumoperitoneum *should not be used in the hypovolemic patient.* Even when the patient appears to be hemodynamically compensated, introduction of pneumoperitoneum can result in sudden decompensation. If a procedure is initiated under pneumoperitoneum and the patient becomes unstable due to ongoing blood loss, the procedure should be immediately converted to a gasless or open approach.

More recent work has emphasized the prevalence of hypercapnia in patients who undergo CO_2 pneumoperitoneum and the adverse cardiovascular effects of increased arterial CO_2 on peripheral vascular tone and myocardial contractility. Acute hypercapnia causes an increase in systemic vascular resistance, a decreased stroke volume, increased heart rate, and decreased cardiac index.[35,42,43] These effects occur even when preload is held constant, and thus must be attributed to the increase in arterial CO_2 rather than a decrease in venous return from pneumoperitoneum.

A final and often overlooked cardiovascular effect of CO_2 pneumoperitoneum is that of increased right-ventricular work. Both through increases in peak airway pressure and by the direct effects of CO_2 on the pulmonary circulation, pulmonary vascular resistance is increased during CO_2 pneumoperitoneum. In patients with normal cardiac function, this is of little consequence. In those with preexisting right-sided cardiac disease, as the consequence of chronic obstructive pulmonary disease, for example, the potential for significant impairment exists.

What is evident from this brief review of recent reports about the cardiovascular effects of CO_2 pneumoperitoneum is that it influences all determinants of cardiac function. Not only can there be diminished preload due to decreases in venous return, but increases in afterload to the right and left ventricle routinely occur, as do decreases in myocardial contractility. All these considerations underline the need for careful preoperative evaluation of patients undergoing CO_2 pneumoperitoneum.

Patients with known cardiac disease are candidates for aggressive intraoperative monitoring, either by Swan–Ganz catheter or continuous transesophageal echo. A rising mean arterial pressure combined with a rising pulse may provide early warning of CO_2-mediated increases in systemic vascular resistance, which in the poorly compensated patient can result in a falling cardiac output.

In the appropriately monitored patient, the administration of intravenous nitroglycerin may reverse these hemodynamic effects. Feig and colleagues[44] placed pulmonary artery catheters in 15 high-risk (ASA III or IV) patients undergoing abdominal procedures via laparoscopy. In 9 of the 15 patients, intraoperative monitoring showed significant changes in cardiac index, systemic vascular resistance, and mean arterial pressure, which returned to baseline following the administration of intravenous nitroglycerin.

Patients should be euvolemic prior to introduction of pneumoperitoneum and volume status should be carefully maintained during surgery. It is especially important that patients do not become hypovolemic intraoperatively, because even if volume is restored, hypotension may persist or recur. In such cases, release of the pneumoperitoneum and conversion to an open technique will be the only means of reestablishing hemodynamic stability.

An awareness of the special cardiac and pulmonary demands imposed by CO_2 pneumoperitoneum will permit the surgeon to adequately evaluate and prepare patients preoperatively and institute suitable intraoperative monitoring in high-risk patients. This will avoid many of the problems that might overtake the patient of an uninformed practitioner. A familiarity of the common manifestations of intraoperative side effects will facilitate rapid recognition and appropriate corrective measures, which should virtually always include immediate discontinuance of CO_2 insufflation and release of pneumoperitoneum until the problem is resolved.

V. CONCLUSION

Enthusiasm for the advantages of laparoscopic surgery must be tempered by an awareness that this new technology brings with it a set of complications unique to the minimally invasive approach. The placement of laparoscopic ports constitutes, in effect, a controlled stab wound to the abdomen. The potential exists for exactly the same types of injuries encountered in the setting of penetrating abdominal trauma, including major hollow and solid visceral trauma and life-threatening vascular injuries. The minimally invasive surgeon should be capable of recognizing such problems as they arise, and facile with their surgical repair. For this reason, if no other, physicians who are not trained surgeons should not be credentialled in laparoscopy. The use of CO_2 pneumoperitoneum results in a variety of hemodymanic sequele resulting from both the mechanical effects of increased intraabdominal pressure and the metabolic effects of CO_2 on the myocardium and peripheral vascular tone. An awareness of these potential hazards as well as the ability to identify and monitor patients at increased risk is essential if complications are to be avoided. This chapter has enumerated the major complications associated with CO_2 pneumoperitoneum and has outlined strategies to avoid such complications, where possible, and deal with the rest as they arise.

REFERENCES

1. Safran DB, Orlando R III: "Physiologic effects of pneumoperitoneum." Am J Surg 1994, 167:281–286.

2. Bongard F, Dubecz S, Klein S: "Complications of therapeutic laparcoscopy." Curr Prob Surg 1994, 31: 868–924.

3. Loffer F, Pent D: "Indications, contraindications, and complications of laparoscopy." Obstet Gynecol Surg 1975, 30(7):407–427.

4. Lieberman BA: "A Clip applicator for laparoscopic sterilization." Fertil Skil 1976, 27(9):1036–1029.

5. Chamberlain G, Brown JC: "Gynaecological laparoscopy: The report of the working party of the confidential enquiry into gynaecological laparoscopy," Royal Coll Obst Gyn, 1978, 165–166.

6. Capelouto CC, Kavoussi LR: "Complications of Laparoscopic surgery." Urology 1993, 42:2–12.

7. Yuzpe, AA: "Pneumoperitoneum needle and trocar injuries in laparoscopy: A survey on possible contributing factors and prevention." J Reprod Med 1990, 35:485–90.

8. Riedel HH, Lehmann-Willenbrock E, Conrad P, et al.: "German pelviscopic statistics for the years 1978–1982." Encoscopy 1986, 18:219–222.

9. Crist DW, Gadacz TR: "Complications of laparoscopic surgery." Surg Clin N Am 1993, 73:265–289.

10. Palmer R: "Safety in laparoscopy." J Reprod Med 1974, 13:1–5.

11. Kent RB: "Subcutaneous emphysema and hypercarbia following laparoscopic cholecystectomy." Arch Surg 1991, 126:1154–1156.

12. Esper E, Russell TE, Coy B, et al.: "Transperitoneal absorption of thermocautery-induced carbon monoxide formation during laparoscopic cholecystectomy." Surg Laparosc Endosc 1994, 4:333–335.

13. Williams MD, Flowers SS, Fenoglio ME, Brown TR: "Richter's hernia following laparoscopy." Surgical Rounds 1995, 18:61–65.

14. Horgan PG, O'Connell PR: "Subumbilical hernia following laparoscopic cholecystectomy." Br J Surg 1993, 80:1595.

15. Thomas AG, McLymont F, Moshipur J.: "Incarcerated hernia after laparoscopic sterilization. A case Report." J Reprod Med 1990; 35:639–40.

16. Fitzgibbons RJ, Jr., Salerno GM, Filipi CJ: "Open laparoscopy." In Zucker, KA (ed.), Surgical Laparoscopy, Chap. 5, St. Louis, MO: Quality Medical Publishing, Inc., 1991.

17. Penfield AJ: "Vascular injuries and their management." In Phillips, JM (ed.), Endoscopy in Gynecology, Chap. 72, Downey, CA: American Association of Gynecologic Laparoscopists, 1978:299–302.

18. Kurzel RB, Edinger DD: "Injury to the great vessels: A hazard of transabdominal endoscopy." South Med J 1983, 76:656–657.

19. Baadsgard SE, Bille S, Egeblad K: "Major vascular injury during gynecologic laparoscopy: report of a case and review of published cases." Acta Obstet Gynecol Scand 1989, 68:283–285.

20. Caprini JA, Swanson J, Coats R, et al.: "The ultrasonic localization of abdominal wall adhesions. Surg. Endosc 1994, 8:245 (Abstract).

21. McDonald PT, Rich NM, Collins, GJ, Jr., et al.: "Vascular trauma secondary to diagnostic and therapeutic procedures: Laparoscopy, Amer J of Surg, 1978, 135:651–655.

22. Penfield, AJ: "Trocar and needle injuries." In Phillips, JM (ed.), *Laparoscopy*, Baltimore, Williams & Wilkins, 1977:236–241.

23. Goss CM (ed): *Gray's Anatomy*. Philadelphia, Lea Febinger, 27th ed, 1959, 684.

24. Salmi A: "Laparoscopic rupture of a patent umbilical vein." Gastrointest Endosc 1986, 32(5):374.

25. Paolaggi JA, Debray C. Accidents de la laparoscopie. Equette nationale. Ann Gastroenterol Hepatol 1976, 12:335–343.

26. Shin CS: "Vascular injury secondary to laparoscopy." NY State J Med [May] 1982; 82(6):935–936.

27. Katz M, Beck P, Tancer ML: "Major vessel injury during laparoscopy: Anatomy of two cases. Am J Obstet Gynecol 1979, 135:544–545.

28. Cohen M: "Hazards of laparoscopy." Arizona Med 1971; 28:830.

29. Jorgensen JO, Lalak NJ, North L, et al.: "Venous stasis during laparoscopic cholecystectomy." Surg Laparosc Endosc 1994; 4:128–133.

30. Jorgensen JO, Gillies RB, Lalak NJ, et al.: "Lower limb venous hemodynamics during laparoscopy: an animal study." Surg Laparosc Endosc 1994, 4:32–35.

31. Millard JA, Hill BB, Cook PS, et al. LH: "Intermittent sequential pneumatic compression in prevention of venous stasis associated with pneumoperitoneum during laparoscopic cholecystectomy." Arch Surg 1993, 128:914–919.

32. Moneta GL, Bedford G, Beach K, et al.: "Duplex ultrasound assessment of venous diameter, peak velocity, and flow patterns." JVS, 1988, 8:286–291.

33. Cali RW.: "Laparoscopy." *Surg Clin N Amer 1980, 60*(2):407–424.

34. Wittgen CM, Andrus CH, Fitzgerald SD, et al.: "Analysis of the hemodynamic and ventilatory effects of laparoscopic cholecystectomy." Arch Surg 1991, 126:997–1001.

35. Hashimoto S, Hashikura Y, Munakata Y, et al.: "Changes in the cardiovascular and respiratory systems during laparoscopic cholecystectomy." J Laparoendosc Surg 1993, 3(6):535–539.

36. Ho HS, Gunther RA, Wolfe BM: "Intraperitoneal carbon dioxide insufflation and cardiopulmonary functions: Laparoscopic cholecystectomy in pigs." Arch Surg 1992; 127:928–933.

37. Scott DB, Julian DG: "Observations on cardiac arrhythmias during laparoscopy." Br Med J 1972; 1:411–413.

38. Beadle EM: "Complications of laparoscopy." In Graber JN, Schultz LS, Pietrafitta JJ, Hickok DF (eds.), Laparoscopic Abdominal Surgery, New York: McGraw Hill, 1993:75–82.

39. Kashtan J, Green JF, Parsons EQ, et al.: "Hemodynamic effects of increased abdominal pressure." *J* Surg Res 1981, 30:249–255.

40. Ishizaki Y, Bandai Y, Shimomura K, et al.: "Changes in splanchnic blood flow and cardiovascular effects following peritoneal insufflation of carbon dioxide." Surg Endosc 1993, 7:420–423.

41. Williams MD, Murr PC: "Laparoscopic insufflation of the abdomen depresses cardiopulmonary function." *Surg Endosc* 1993, 7:12–16.

42. Ho HS, Saunders CJ, Corso FA, et al.: "The effects of CO$_2$ pneumoperitoneum on hemodynamics in hemorrhaged animals." Surgery 1993, 114(2):381–388.

43. Westerband A, Van DeWater JM, Amzallag M, et al.: "Cardiovascular changes during laparoscopic cholecystectomy." *Surg Gynecol Obstet* 1992; 175:535–538.

44. Feig BW, Berger DH, Dougherty TB, et al.: "Pharmacologic intervention can reestablish baseline hemodynamic parameters during laparoscopy." Surgery 1994, 116:733–741.

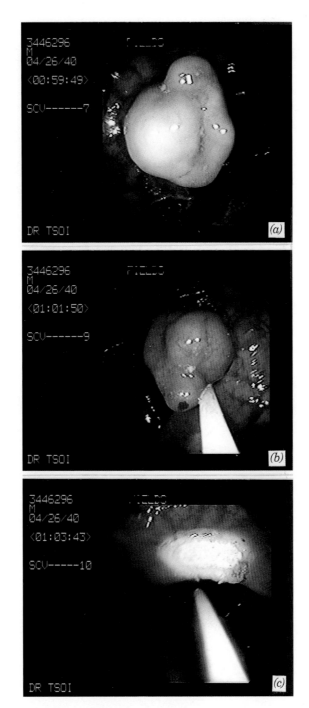

Figure 1.1. (*a*) Polyp identified during colonoscopy; (*b*) polypectomy with a snare; (*c*) cauterized mucosal surface after polypectomy.

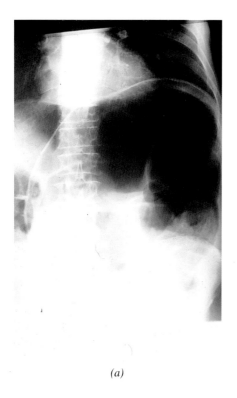

(a)

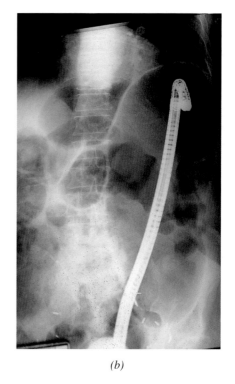

(b)

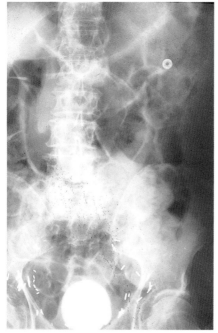

(c)

Figure 1.2. (*a*) Sigmoid volvulus seen on plain abdominal radiography; (*b*) reduction of volvulus with a flexible endoscope; (*c*) postreduction film.

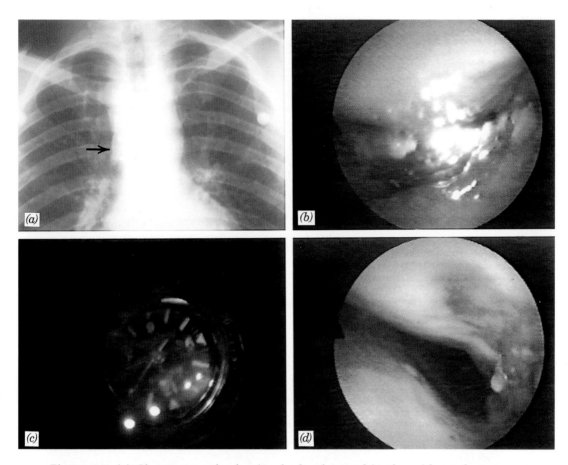

Figure 1.3. (*a*) Chest x-ray of a foreign body observed in the mid esophagus; (*b*) foreign body is confirmed by esophagoscopy; (*c*) the foreign body (a wrist watch) removed via esophagoscopy; (*d*) superficial mucosal ulceration after foreign body removal.

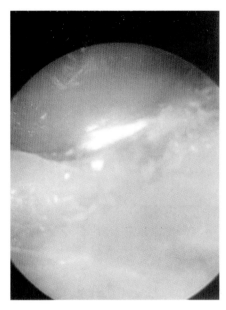

Figure 1.5. Retroperitoneal dissection using the dissecting balloon. The retroperitoneal space is carefully entered between the peritoneum and the retroperitoneum. The filmy area at the center of the picture is the retroperitoneal space being exposed by the dissecting balloon.

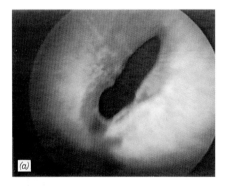 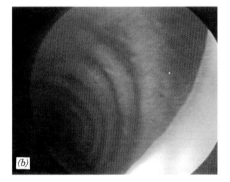

Figure 4.3. (*a*) Diaphragmatic laceration seen during trauma laparoscopy (courtesy of E. K. M. Tsoi). (*b*) Laparoscopic view of the thoracic cavity through the diaphragmatic laceration.

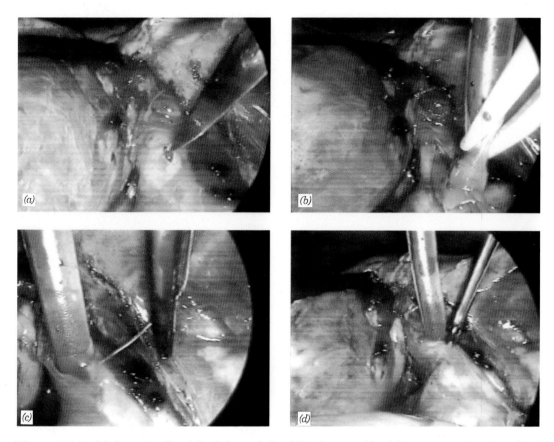

Figure 7.21. (*a*) Longitudinal incision of the bile duct wall with a conventional scalpel. (*b*) Insertion of a T-tube into the common bile duct. (*c*) Placement of a ski-needle through the bile duct wall. (*d*) Closure of choledochotomy with an extracorporeally interlaced knot.

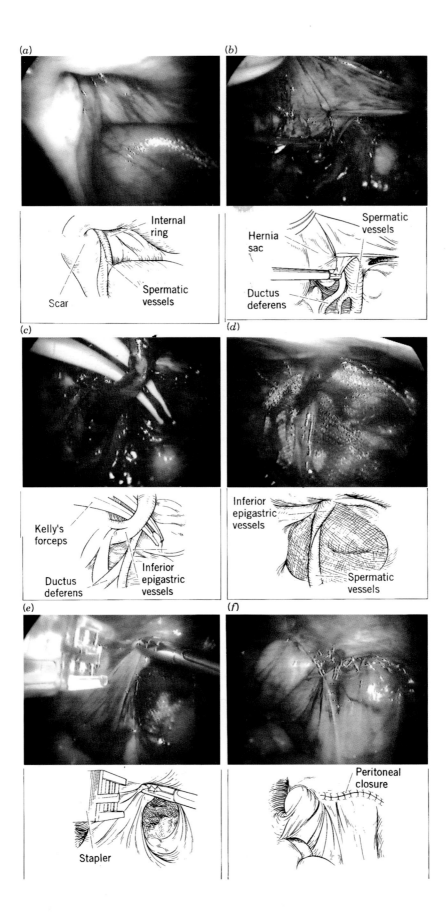

(a)

Internal
ring

Spermatic
vessels

Scar

(b)

Spermatic
vessels

Hernia
sac

Ductus
deferens

(c)

Kelly's
forceps

Ductus
deferens

Inferior
epigastric
vessels

(d)

Inferior
epigastric
vessels

Spermatic
vessels

(e)

Stapler

(f)

Peritoneal
closure

Figure 7.25. TAPP hernioplasty for right recurrent indirect inguinal hernia with the subcutaneous lift system. (*a*) Laparoscopic view of the internal inguinal ring. (*b*) Dissection of the hernia sac around the internal ring. (*c*) Dissection of the inferior epigastric vessels. (*d*) Placement of the mesh. (*e*) Closure of the peritoneum over the mesh with a stapler. (*f*) Completion of the hernia repair.

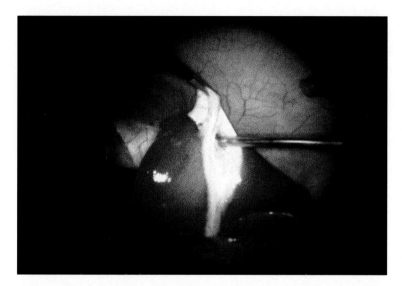

Figure 8.4. Cholecystectomy with a planar lifting allows conventional instruments, such as Babcock clamps demonstrated here, to be used during laparoscopic dissection.

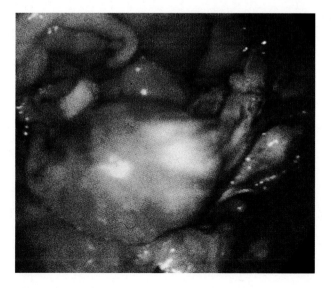

Figure 8.5. A view of the uterus during laparoscopic-assisted vaginal hysterectomy utilizing planar lifting.

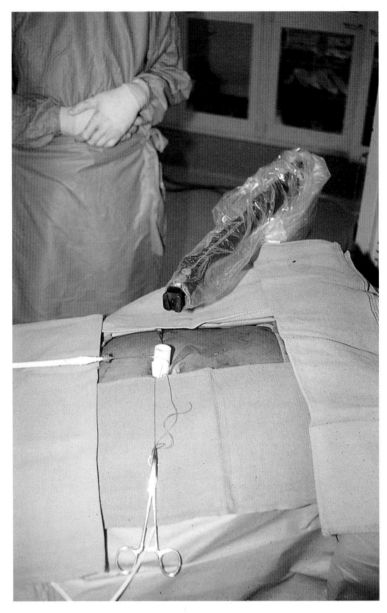

Figure 9.1. The telescopic arm of the abdominal wall lifter covered with a sterile drape is placed into the sterile field.

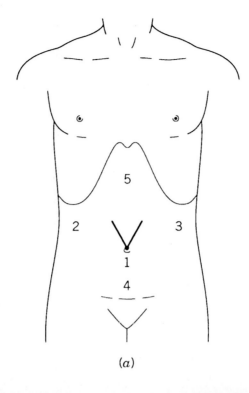

(a)

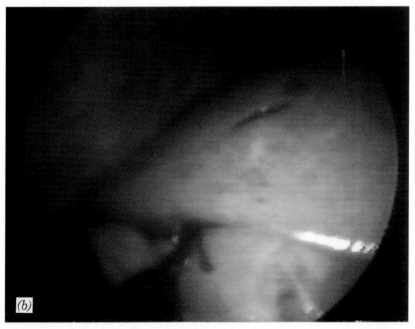

(b)

Figure 9.2. (a) Diamond-shaped access placement for diagnostic laparoscopy. Access number 5 can be omitted for limited pelvic peritoneoscopy. (b) Liver laceration caused by stabbing identified during trauma laparoscopy.

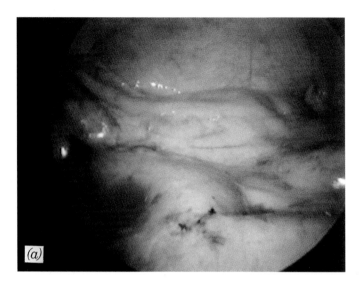

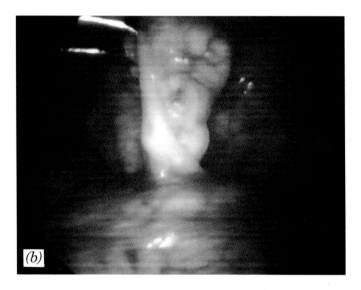

Figure 9.3. (*a*) Small bowel laceration was identified during diagnostic laparoscopy and placed back into the abdomen after repaired extracorporeally with silk sutures. (*b*) A normal appendix is being examined with the help of an Allis clamp.

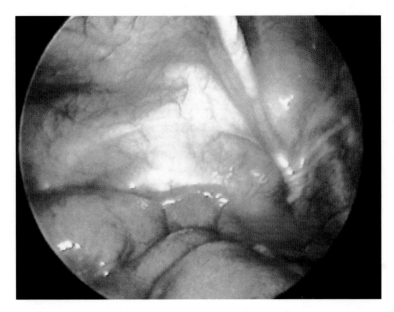

Figure 9.5. Purulent drainage noted in the abdomen of a patient with HIV disease and nonspecific abdominal pain.

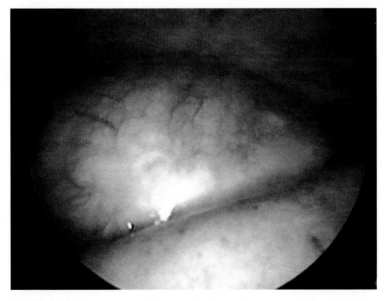

Figure 9.6. Ischemic cecum with purulent exudate noted during diagnostic laparoscopy.

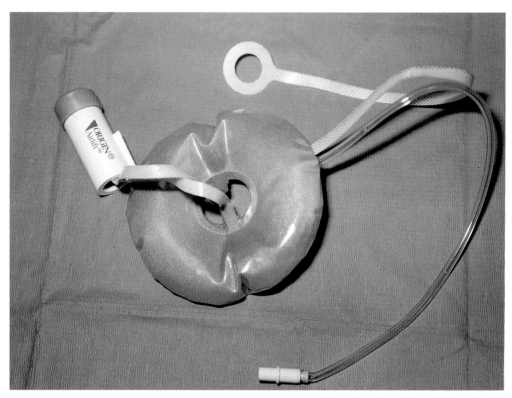

Figure 9.7. Picture of the inflatable abdominal wall lifter—Airlift® .

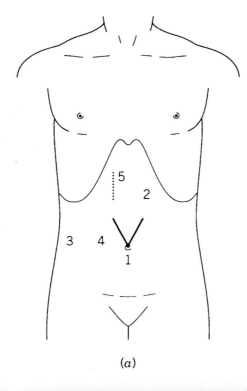

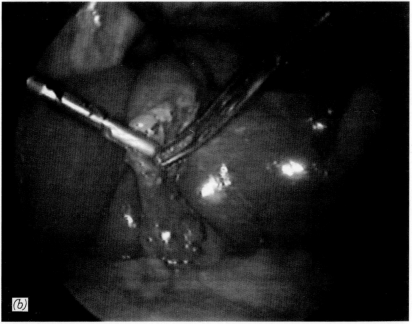

Figure 9.8. (*a*) Diagram showing access for laparoscopic cholecystectomy. Access 5 is a miniparamedian incision used for choledochoscopy and suturing of the choledochus. (*b*) Isolation of the cystic duct of an inflamed gallbladder using a tonsil clamp.

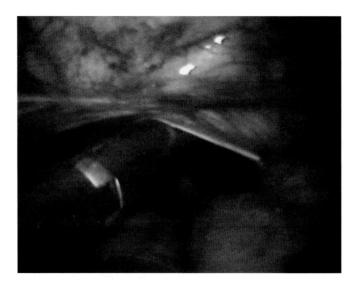

Figure 9.11. Gastric volvulus in the hiatal hernia is being reduced back into the abdomen with an endoscopic grasper.

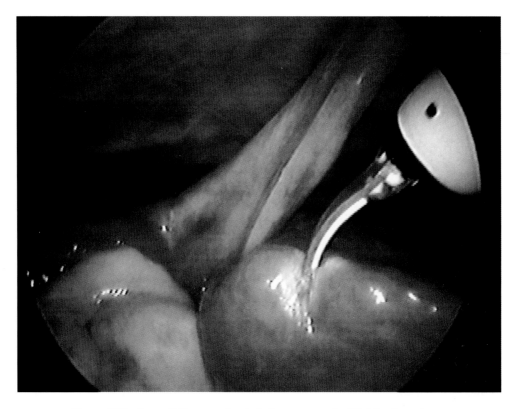

Figure 9.13. A small liver wedge is being removed with bipolar scissors.

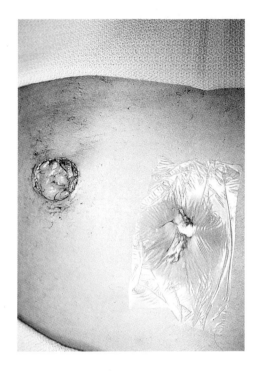

Figure 9.16. Picture of a patient who has laparoscopic sigmoid colostomy.

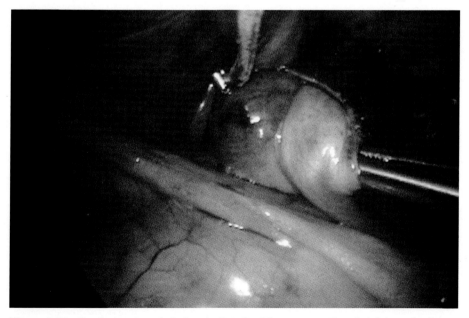

Figure 9.19. Cord structure is being isolated with a conventional right-angle clamp.

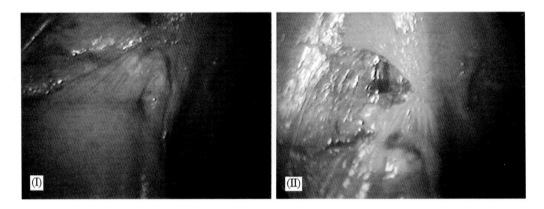

Figure 9.20. (I) A CAPD patient who has been diagnosed to have peritoneal fibrosis during laparoscopy. (II) Thick fibrous tissue was partially removed with endoscopic instruments.

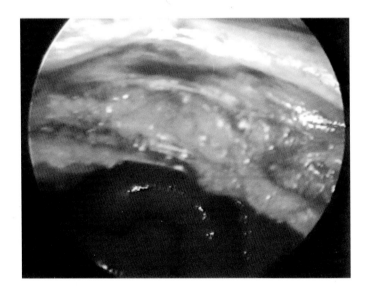

Figure 11.1. A small incision is made for placement of an Army–Navy retractor and a video-laparoscope at the beginning of exploratory laparotomy.

7

SUBCUTANEOUS LIFT SYSTEM (SCLS) FOR LAPAROSCOPIC SURGERY

Hideo Nagai, M.D.

I. INTRODUCTION

Abdominal-wall lift eliminates all the complications associated with blind puncture by needles and trocars, insufflation with CO_2, and high intraabdominal pressure. It also enables laparoscopic surgeons to perform sophisticated procedures using conventional instruments and techniques for suturing, tying, unlimited suction, and lavish irrigation.[1] Some surgeons have called this new method of abdominal access "gasless" or "without pneumoperitoneum".[2-4] Nagai and his colleagues used the phrase "without pneumoperitoneum" in their original abstract.[5] The wall lift, however, actually does cause pneumoperitoneum because it allows air to enter the abdominal cavity. Thus it might be said that abdominal-wall lift provides "passive"

Abdominal Access in Open and Laparoscopic Surgery
Edited by Edmund K. M. Tsoi and Claude H. Organ, Jr.
ISBN 0-471-13352-3 Copyright © 1996 by Wiley-Liss, Inc.

pneumoperitoneum, while gas insufflation creates "active" pneumoperitoneum.

Even during the early developmental stages of laparoscopic cholecystectomy, the concept of abdominal-wall lift was explored to find a method that allowed better exposure and more dexterous performance of procedures that might be too complex to do under peritoneal insufflation. Mouret seems to have been the first surgeon to have conceived of such a device.[6] His apparatus, called a "suspenseur de paroi," consists of a curved rod with a triangular shape that is inserted into the abdominal cavity and pulled upward with a row of chains. Gazayerli and associates reported a similar T-shaped instrument that assisted in obtaining better visualization in laparoscopic colectomy for obese patients.[7] These devices were used in combination with CO_2 gas either after establishing pneumoperitoneum or while maintaining intraabdominal pressure from inside. Hence, the complications associated with CO_2 insufflation still persisted.

Laparoscopic cholecystectomy without auxiliary gas insufflation was first conducted by the author and colleagues in January 1991 with the use of a subcutaneous lift system (SCLS).[5] This method utilizes physiologic adhesion of the subcutaneous tissue between the skin and the underlying fascia and muscle layers. One of the advantages of SCLS over full-thickness wall lift from inside the peritoneal cavity, as designed by Mouret and Gazayerli or lately produced by Origin Medsystems, USA, is its applicability in all patients regardless of past history of abdominal surgery or unexpected adhesion in the peritoneal cavity. Another positive feature of SCLS is the elimination of painful and adhesion-prone traumas to the peritoneum that are unavoidable in full-thickness wall-lift systems.

II. SUBCUTANEOUS LIFT SYSTEM (SCLS)

Two systems for subcutaneous-wall lift are available on the Japanese market: one developed by the authors and the other by Hashimoto and his colleagues (Figure 7.1).[1,4] The former is being manufactured by Mizuho Ika Co. and the latter by Takasago Ika Co., both located in Tokyo. Hashimoto's method uses a pair of thick wires (3 mm in diameter) to form a triangular plane, whereas our SCLS utilizes 2–3 parallel thin wires (1.0–1.2 mm in diameter). This chapter describes the author's SCLS.

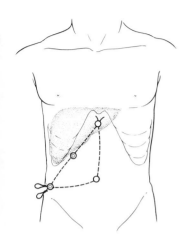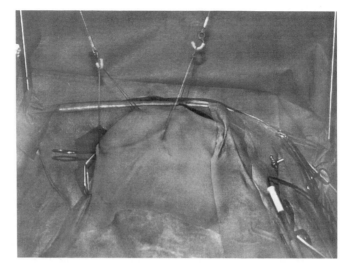

Figure 7.1. Hashimoto's subcutaneous lift method. Two thick wires are inserted into the subcutaneous tissue of the right upper abdominal quadrant to form a triangle. The triangular plane is then pulled upwards with winching devices using twines. Courtesy of Dr. D. Hashimoto.

III. INSTRUMENTS

Lifting Handles and Bar

The arms of a lifting handle are attached to both ends of a Kirschner wire advanced through the skin and subcutaneous tissue (Figures 7.2 and 7.3). The skin tolerates the upward traction very well, while the fascia seems to be susceptible to laceration.

The handle is raised toward the L-shaped bar by means of a small winching device. The lifting bar is securely fixed onto the rail of the operating table. The lifting bar is foldable and becomes compact, thus facilitating sterilization.

Sheaths

A 140- × 11-mm sheath (Figure 7.4) is used to insert the laparoscope, which can be fixed firmly or semifirmly along with the sheath by a self-retracting device called a Laparo-Hand (Mizuho Ika Co., Tokyo), attached to the arm of the lifting bar (Figure 7.5). Use of sheath-mediated compression avoids any damage

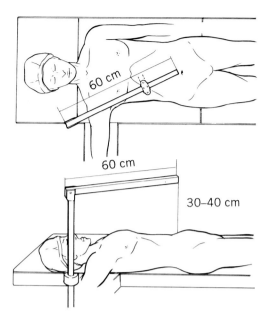

Figure 7.2. The position of the lifting bar. The tip of its 60 cm-long arm should be placed 30–40 cm over the umbilicus.

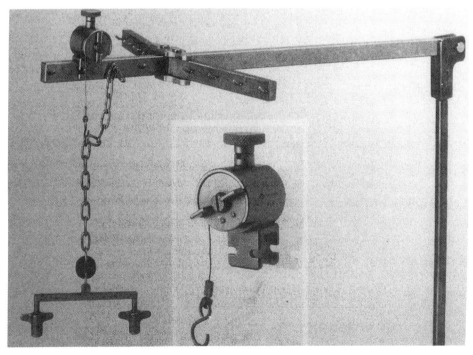

Figure 7.3. The lifting handle attached to the arm of the lifting bar. A small winching device helps raise the abdominal wall.

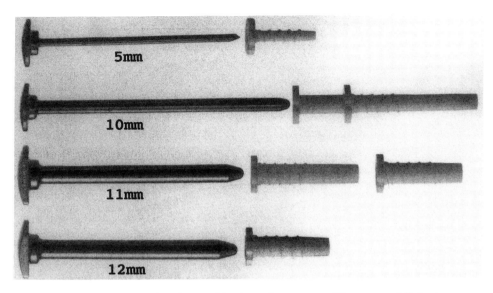

Figure 7.4. Trocars and sheaths used in the subcutaneous lift system. All the trocars except those 5 mm wide have blunt tips. They are inserted into the abdominal cavity after trocar sites have been opened, as with open laparoscopy at the umbilicus or with tips of forceps below the xiphoid process. Blunt insertion lessens the risk of bleeding from the muscular layers of the abdominal wall.

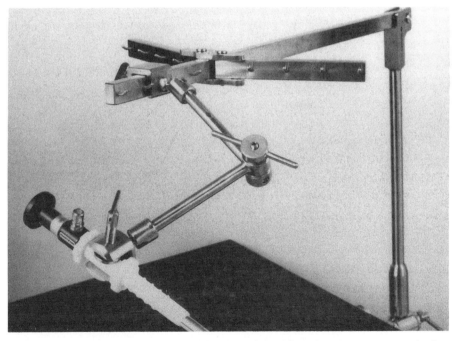

Figure 7.5. Laparo-Hand attached to the arm of the lifting bar. It compresses the laparoscope indirectly through the sheath so as to avoid mechanical damage to the shaft of the instrument.

103

to the shaft of the laparoscope; in contrast, direct seizure without a sheath by other self-retractors used for insufflation systems will cause damage to the shaft of the laparoscope.

For manipulating instruments, sheaths 60 to 80 mm long and 6 or 11 mm wide are placed in the abdominal wall. The sheaths are inserted into the abdominal cavity with trocars.

Because all these sheaths can be airtight and securely adapted to corresponding SurgiPorts (U.S. Surgical Corporation, USA) or other trocar sheaths used with "active" pneumoperitoneum, our abdominal-wall lift method can be quickly and easily converted to or combined with the pneumoperitoneum.

Ancillary Instruments

All of the laparoscopic instruments used for conventional peritoneal insufflation can also be utilized in SCLS. In addition, instruments similar to those used in conventional open surgery can be employed. Especially useful are modified Metzenbaum scissors (Figure 7.6) and modified Kelly clamps (Figure 7.7). The distance between the tip and pivot of the instruments is 80 to 100 mm. When connected to an electrocautery system, these insulated Kelly clamps help not only to dissect tissue but also to coagulate vessels.

An electrode combined with a suction tube (Figure 7.8) is another useful instrument for simultaneous hemostasis and suction of blood. A gas-insufflation system might not support the application of such an instrument.

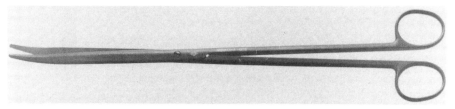

Figure 7.6. Metzenbaum scissors utilized in the subcutaneous lift system. The length between the tip and pivot of the instrument is 8–10 cm.

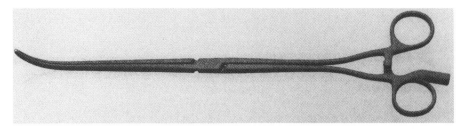

Figure 7.7. Forceps based on Kelly forceps. The instrument is designed to have a wide grip and a safe insulation system that allows connection to an electrocautery system.

IV. PROCEDURES

Cholecystectomy

Using open laparoscopy (Figure 7.9), an 11-mm sheath combined with a trocar is inserted into the abdominal cavity through an incision in the infraumbilical area. Only the sheath is left behind for the insertion of the laparoscope. Two Kirschner wires are placed just beneath the skin rather than through all layers of the abdominal wall, one in the upper portion of the umbilicus and the other at the right costal margin. The wires are attached to the lifting handles and pulled upward.

The umbilical wire and handle should be as close to the laparoscope as possible. If placed immediately above the umbilicus, the laparoscope has the greatest look-down angle, and in some cases the angle is greater than that obtained with active pneumoperitoneum (Figure 7.10). The costal wire and handle should be long enough to sufficiently elevate the costal margin. For an

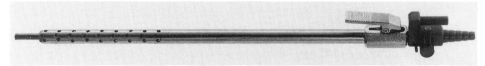

Figure 7.8. Suction-tube electrode. The tube gets sheathed or unsheathed in a one-touch operation without being pulled out of the abdominal cavity. The body of the suction system is insulated except at the tip of the tube. One can coagulate a bleeding point with this tube while employing suction. See Figure 7.19.

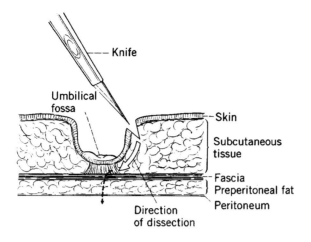

Knife

Umbilical fossa

Skin

Subcutaneous tissue

Fascia
Preperitoneal fat
Peritoneum

Direction of dissection

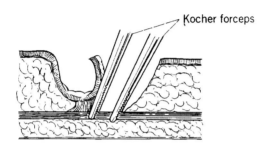

Kocher forceps

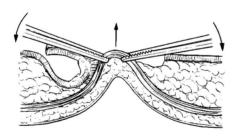

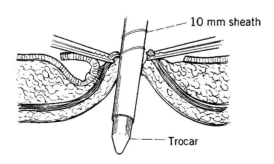

10 mm sheath

Trocar

Figure 7.9. Technique of open laparoscopy at the umbilicus. One should dissect the subcutaneous tissue toward the bottom of the umbilicus. The fascia in the periumbilical region can be brought upward to the level of the skin even in obese patients under adequate anesthesia with muscle relaxation.

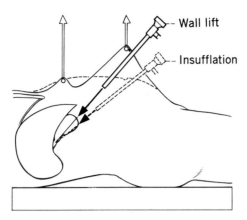

Figure 7.10. Difference of the angle of the laparoscope in the subcutaneous lift system and in the insufflation method. The look-down angle might be greater in the lift system than in the insufflation method due to the raised insertion site of the laparoscope.

obese patient, a third wire and handle is anchored on the lower part of the anterior chest wall (Figure 7.11).

With elevation of the abdominal wall, air flows into the abdominal cavity through the umbilical sheath (passive pneumoperitoneum). A laparoscope is then inserted through the sheath. Sheaths for manipulating are placed under laparoscopic vision. One should realize that the trocar sites for manipulation differ in SCLS from those used for active pneumoperitoneum. To avoid inter-

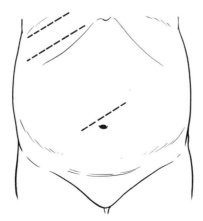

Figure 7.11. Position of wires for cholecystectomy in an obese patient. A third wire should be placed above the right costal margin.

ference of the instruments with each other, sheaths for the manipulating instruments should be arranged so that they are aligned as perpendicular as possible to the axis of the laparoscope (Figure 7.12). Especially important is the location of the sheath below the xiphoid process. The xiphoid sheath, 11 mm in
diameter, should be placed obliquely through the attachment of the hepatic
falciform ligament toward Calot's triangle at approximately 45° to the horizontal plane (Figure 7.13). An upright position is to be avoided so that the arm of
the lifting bar does not stand in the way. One should determine the site and direction of the xiphoid sheath after a trial puncture with a fine needle for identification of the needle tip viewed through the laparoscope.

Two auxiliary 5-mm sheaths are placed on the mid-axillary line of the
right flank instead of in the anterior abdominal wall as with insufflation (Figures 7.12 and 7.14).

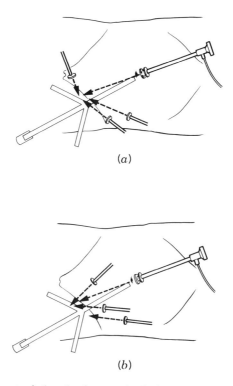

(a)

(b)

Figure 7.12. Placement of sheaths for manipulating instruments. The directions of
the instruments should be as perpendicular as possible to the axis of the laparoscope, as in (a). Parallel positioning of the instruments increases the possible interference of the instruments with each other, as in (b).

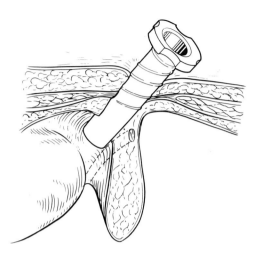

Figure 7.13. Direction of the xiphoid sheath. The sheath should be placed obliquely to appear on the right plane of the falciform ligament. One must take care not to penetrate the left side of the ligament.

Cholecystectomy is done in the same way as with the peritoneal insufflation method. If the laparoscope is held semifirmly with the above-mentioned Laparo-Hand, the surgery can be performed by two doctors without a cameraman. The surgeon, standing on the patient's left side, manipulates dissecting and cutting instruments through the xiphoid sheath with the right hand, while he or she handles the laparoscope with the left hand for focusing and changing views. The semifixed scope stays still even after the surgeon releases his or her grip. Thus, the laparoscope can serve as the surgeon's voluntary eye, not the cameraman's.

The assistant on the patient's right side holds two 5-mm graspers, one with each hand. The handles of the graspers should be directed upward so as not to touch the operating table or the patient's body (Figure 7.15). The graspers, introduced from the flank, should be handled like a lever to pull only the tissue by the tip, up or down. At the beginning of dissection of Calot's triangle, it is advised that the assistant raise the neck of the gallbladder high enough with the right grasper and push down the duodenum with the closed tip of the left grasper (Figure 7.16).

Intraoperative cholangiography can be done easily. The surgeon simply inserts a catheter of any type through the xiphoid sheath. The tube is held in place with the grooved and curved tips of the forceps (Figure 7.17). These tips

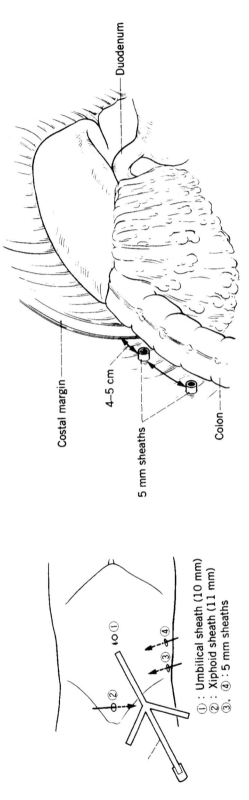

Figure 7.14. Placement of two 5 mm sheaths in the right flank. They should be placed as laterally as possible, just above the level of the colon and the omentum.

Duodenum

Costal margin

4–5 cm

5 mm sheaths

Colon

① : Umbilical sheath (10 mm)
② : Xiphoid sheath (11 mm)
③, ④ : 5 mm sheaths

110

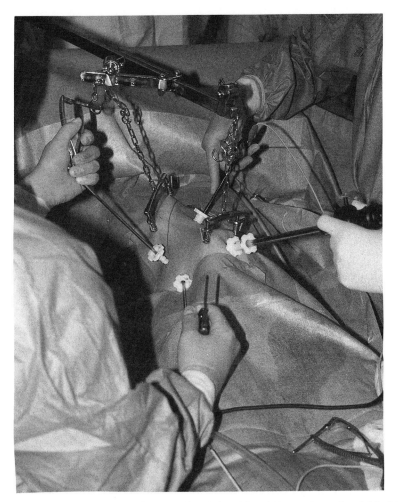

Figure 7.15. The assistant standing on the right side of the patient should hold the graspers with their handles directed upward to avoid "collision" with the operating table or the patient's body.

can facilitate insertion into the cystic duct. Our success rate for cholangiography amounts to 99%.

Using SCLS, dissection of the gallbladder from the liver bed may be done with a conventional cautery (Figure 7.18). Coagulation of any bleeding points becomes easy with an insulated suction tube connected to an electrocoagulation device (Figure 7.19). Both infusion and suction of a large volume of saline

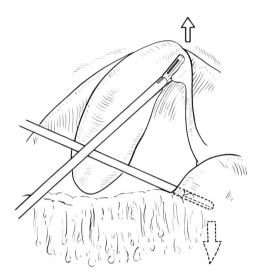

Figure 7.16. Advised technique of the assistant to visualize Calot's triangle. The right grasper should raise the neck of the gallbladder, while the left one pushes down the duodenum with its closed tip.

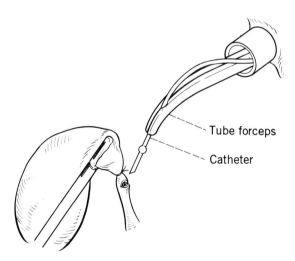

Tube forceps

Catheter

Figure 7.17. Insertion of a catheter through the xiphoid sheath for intraoperative cholangiography.

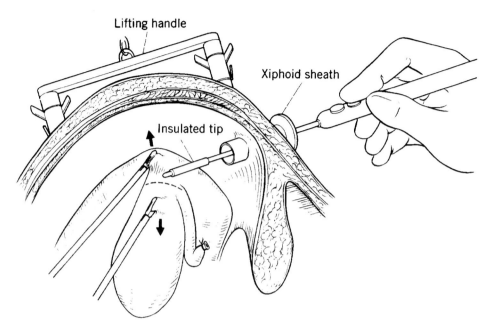

Figure 7.18. Dissection of the gallbladder from the liver bed using a conventional electrode.

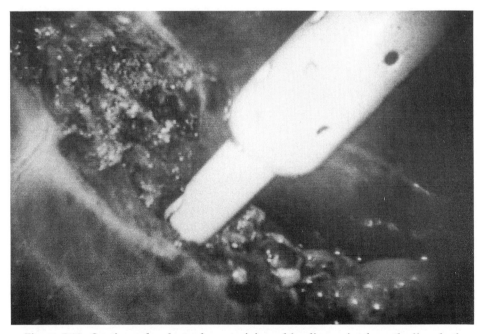

Figure 7.19. Suction-tube electrode cauterizing a bleeding point from the liver bed.

can be quite easily done in a very short time without degrading the laparoscopic view (Figure 7.20). Thorough irrigation of the operative field and clearance of blood clots remarkably reduce pain after surgery.

A large amount of air causes discomfort for several days postoperatively. Therefore, the abdominal cavity should be filled with 500 ml of saline to remove as much air as possible before closing the wounds. If this procedure is followed, postoperative pain is minimal, and almost all patients can walk the next day.

Three hundred and forty-seven patients with cholecystolithiasis or gallbladder polyps have undergone laparoscopic cholecystectomy with SCLS at our institution and affiliated hospitals. A total of 343 patients were managed successfully utilizing only SCLS. In three cases of the earlier series (nos. 6, 11, and 14), SCLS was combined with the insufflation method due to difficulty in obtaining a good field of vision. One patient with morbid obesity [case no. 123 of the series: female, 151 cm (60 in), 87 kg (182 lbs)] could not be managed with SCLS and had to be converted to insufflation.

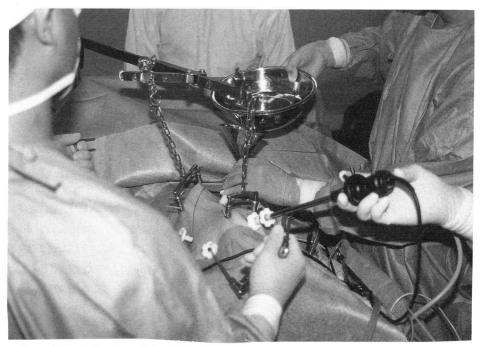

Figure 7.20. Irrigation of the abdominal cavity with a large volume of saline poured through a funnel.

In two of the 347 cases (0.5%), we converted the laparoscopic procedure to open surgery due to bleeding and severe adhesion in Calot's triangle. Two patients with cirrhosis of the liver had postoperative bleeding that required open surgery for hemostasis. No deaths occurred. Therefore, in this series, there was a 0% mortality rate and 0.5% incidence of severe morbidity.

Very few patients complained of pain or tenderness at the lift sites. More than half of the patients required no postoperative analgesics. Pain came mostly from small incisions at the umbilicus and below the xiphoid, the same pain encountered with insufflation.

Choledocholithotomy

Strategy for treatment of common bile-duct stones still remains controversial. The authors maintain that bile-duct stones should be treated laparoscopically with the same options as in open surgery. First, we try to extract common bile-duct stones via the cystic duct with the help of a small-caliber choledochoscope. If unsuccessful in transcystic duct exploration, we then incise the common bile duct and remove the stones with a spoon, forceps, balloon, or basket with or without choledochoscopic guidance. After choledochotomy the bile-duct wall is closed primarily without a T-tube if we are certain that no stone remains. If we are not certain, we insert a T-tube and suture the incised wall with a few absorbable sutures. We have not routinely performed pre- or postoperative endoscopic papillotomy for stone extraction because of the lack of specialized staff and for fear of possible complications from the endoscopic treatment.

The reason for this strategy in laparoscopic surgery is that we are in the process of adopting SCLS, which is a system that allows us to extract bile-duct stones, insert a T-tube, and suture the incision much more easily than with an insufflation system (Figure 7.21). This ease results not only from not needing to take care of gas leakage, but also from the availability of more sophisticated instruments. Of special note is a sliding tube for introducing a fiber-optic choledochoscope through the xiphoid sheath (Figure 7.22). Since air-tightness is not required, smooth to-and-fro movement of the scope is facilitated. We also have designed a special needle holder for suturing in SCLS. This holder has a curved tip that provides more options for the direction of a needle than does a straight holder used with insufflation (Figure 7.23).

SCLS has been attempted in 27 patients with choledocholithiasis. Two patients were treated with transcystic duct removal of common bile-duct

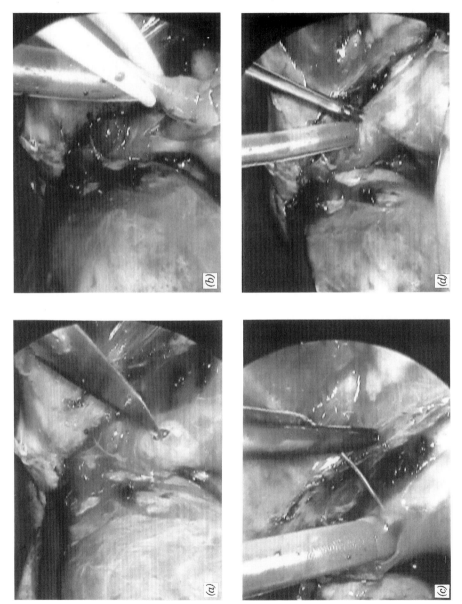

Figure 7.21. (*a*) Longitudinal incision of the bile duct wall with a conventional scalpel. (*b*) Insertion of a T-tube into the common bile duct. (*c*) Placement of a ski-needle through the bile duct wall. (*d*) Closure of choledochotomy with an extracorporeally interlaced knot. (See insert for color representation.)

116

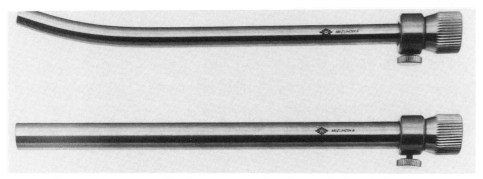

Figure 7.22. Sliding tubes for insertion of a fiber-optic choledochoscope.

stones and one with preoperative endoscopic papillotomy was followed by laparoscopic cholecystectomy. In the remaining 24 patients, laparoscopic choledochotomy was performed and bile-duct stones were successfully extracted with either a basket or a Fogarty catheter under visualization with a fiber-optic choledochoscope. T-tube drainage was performed in 23 patients. In 21 of these patients, a T-tube was inserted into the common bile duct under laparoscopic guidance and the incised duct wall was sealed with one to three in-

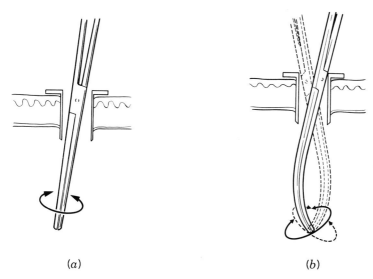

(a)   (b)

Figure 7.23 Needle holders, straight (a) and curved (b). A curved holder has a wider range of movement than a straight one.

terrupted sutures. In two patients of the earlier series of bile duct stones (nos. 1 and 12), minilaparotomy was combined for insertion of a T-tube and suture of the choledochotomy after laparoscopic choledocholithotomy. One patient underwent choledochotomy plus primary suture of the bile-duct incision. No mortality or severe morbidity was encountered.

Hernia Repair

Inguinal hernia repair by SCLS is possible with either a transabdominal preperitoneal approach (TAPP) or extraperitoneal access (EP). The authors have performed 18 cases of laparoscopic hernioplasty with SCLS, 15 with TAPP, and three with EP (Tables 7.1 and 7.2). We did not use any other special instruments than those used for SCLS cholecystectomy, except a sheet of mesh and a hernia stapler.

Although spinal or epidural anesthesia seems feasible in hernioplasty with SCLS, general anesthesia with tracheal intubation may be better during the initial experience with this procedure because of the length of the operation. If the surgeon becomes confident enough to perform hernioplasty in less

TABLE 7.1

Hernioplasty with SCLS

Indirect (recurrence 2)	14
Direct (recurrence 2)	4
Total	18

TABLE 7.2

Approach and anesthesia in laparoscropic hernioplasty with SCLS

Transabdominal + general anesthesia	13
Transabdominal + spinal	2
Extraabdominal + spinal	1
Extraabdominal + epidural	2
Total	18

than an hour, spinal anesthesia may then be used. In our series, 13 patients underwent general anesthesia and five local (spinal and epidural) anesthesia.

Transabdominal Preperitoneal (TAPP) Access. The surgeon stands

on the contralateral side, the assistant on the ipsilateral side of the hernia (Figure 7.24). Open laparoscopy is performed in the upper portion of the umbilicus. After insertion of the laparoscope, two sets of Kirschner wires and lifting handles are placed in the abdominal wall, one wire just below the umbilicus and the other 3–4 cm cranial to the ipsilateral inguinal ligament. As the handles are raised toward the arm of the lifting bar and the patient is tilted at approximately 15–20° with the head down, a good view of the inguinal floor is provided.

A 12-mm sheath and a 5-mm sheath are placed in the abdominal wall on the contralateral side for manipulation by the surgeon. A 5-mm sheath is inserted on the ipsilateral side through which the assistant introduces a grasper.

The operative techniques used in TAPP are exactly the same as those used with pneumoperitoneum (Figure 7.25): incision of the peritoneum around the internal inguinal ring, then dissection of the hernia sac followed by exposure of the transversalis fascia, vas deferens (uterine round ligament), in-

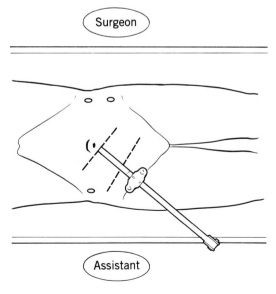

Figure 7.24. Position of the surgeon, the assistant, the lifting bar, and the trocar sites for right inguinal hernioplasty.

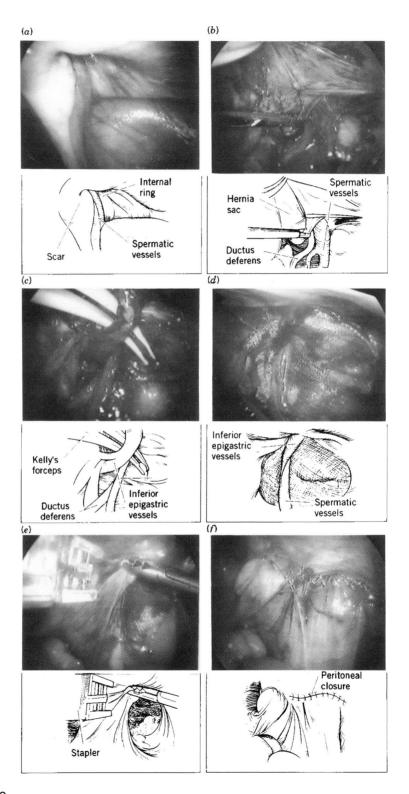

(a)

Internal ring

Scar

Spermatic vessels

(b)

Spermatic vessels

Hernia sac

Ductus deferens

(c)

Kelly's forceps

Ductus deferens

Inferior epigastric vessels

(d)

Inferior epigastric vessels

Spermatic vessels

(e)

Stapler

(f)

Peritoneal closure

ternal spermatic vessels, iliopubic tract, and Cooper ligament. An adequately large sheet of polypropylene mesh is attached to these structures and fixed with a hernia stapler to the transversalis fascia, iliopubic tract, and Cooper ligament. Care must be taken to avoid any injury to nerves, especially to the lateral femoral cutaneous nerve and ilioinguinal nerve. The incised peritoneum may be repaired with staples, but it can also be managed with a running suture, which does not require a time-consuming procedure so long as SCLS is adopted.

Extraperitoneal (EP) Access. Instruments, sites of wall lift, and the patient's position are identical to those in TAPP. A small skin and fascia incision below the umbilicus provides access both to the space anterior to the posterior lamina of rectus sheath and to the preperitoneal space below the linea arcuata toward the pubic symphysis. The working space can be conveniently established with a balloon dissector (PBD, Origin Medsystems, USA), but blunt dissection with a finger, a round-tipped rod, or even the laparoscope itself can also suffice. Inadvertent perforation of the peritoneum incurs elevation of this area and sometimes prolapse of the intestine into the operative field. As the preperitoneal space enlarges with further dissection, the peritoneum usually goes down even if lacerations have occurred. If the peritoneum does not go down, a fan-shaped retractor inserted from under the scope will help depress the bulging tissues and organs.

Dissection of the preperitoneal space should be started on the assistant's (ipsilateral) side because a scissors or a rod inserted and manipulated by the assistant through the first sheath on this side greatly helps the surgeon obtain a space large enough to introduce a 12-mm sheath on the contralateral side. As mentioned earlier in the description of cholecystectomy, sheaths for instruments should be placed at a large angle to the axis of the scope to avoid mutual interference.

Care must be taken to avoid injury of any incarcerated viscera during dissection and division of the hernia sac from the inguinal canal. One should

Figure 7.25. TAPP hernioplasty for right recurrent indirect inguinal hernia with the subcutaneous lift system. (*a*) Laparoscopic view of the internal inguinal ring. (*b*) Dissection of the hernia sac around the internal ring. (*c*) Dissection of the inferior epigastric vessels. (*d*) Placement of the mesh. (*e*) Closure of the peritoneum over the mesh with a stapler. (*f*) Completion of the hernia repair. (See insert for color representation.)

open the sac when uncertain of its contents. If the sac is large enough, it can be pulled out of the body to be incised and examined as in the conventional open anterior approach (Figure 7.26). Repair with mesh is the same as in TAPP.

Bowel Resection

Our initial application of SCLS for bowel resection has posed a problem that still prevents its wide use. The major obstacle is the limited movement afforded by the laparoscope and the camera. Laparoscopic surgery for colon cancer requires frequent and wide-ranging motion to obtain an adequate view of the operative field. For example, when we perform a laparoscopic or laparoscope-assisted resection of moderately advanced sigmoid colon cancer, the origin of the inferior mesenteric artery is identified and divided and the left lateral peritoneal reflection of the descending colon and the mesentery of the rectosigmoid colon are mobilized. This means that the laparoscope's position must constantly be changed from cranial to caudal, or from upright to horizontal, and vice versa. The arm of the lifting bar tends to get in the way and inhibit such rapid repositioning.

For resection of a benign lesion or an early cancer of the small intestine, the ileocecal region, the transverse colon, or the sigmoid colon, SCLS is an ex-

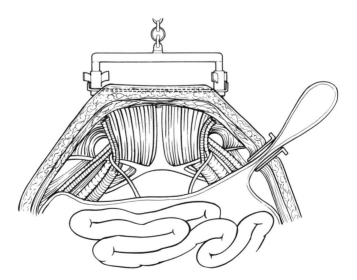

Figure 7.26. Extraperitoneal approach for inguinal hernia. A large hernia sac can be treated extracorporeally, as done in the conventional open method, without using an automatic suture device.

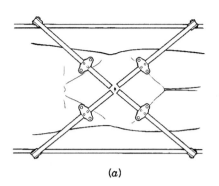 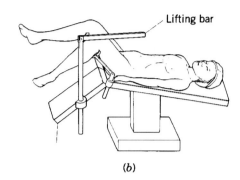

Lifting bar

(a)   (b)

Figure 7.27. Position of the lifting bar for colectomy. The position should be changed according to the site of the lesion (a). For intracorporeal anastomosis, as after resection of the lower part of the sigmoid colon, the patient should be placed in the lithotomy position in advance with the lifting bar attached to a rail on the left lower limb of the operating table (b).

cellent access to treatment (Figure 7.27). Although the ease of SCLS in suturing and tying lends itself to the performance of sophisticated techniques, it might be advisable to perform anastomosis of the colon extracorporeally. The double-stapling technique can be applied after resection of a lesion in the rectosigmoid colon. The small intestine may be reconstructed intracorporeally with a functional end-to-end anastomosis (Figure 7.28).

Gynecologic Procedures

Some Japanese gynecologists are enthusiastically welcoming SCLS for pelvic surgery. Isaka and associates of Tokyo have performed laparoscope-assisted vaginal hysterectomy (LAVH) with SCLS and describe its advantages over gas insufflation, citing the merit that the wall-lift system does not block the view of the operative field even if the pelvic cavity joins with the vagina.[9] They have modified our system by placing a single Kirschner wire instead of two horizontal wires in the subcutaneous tissue on the median line of the lower abdomen (Figure 7.29). They claim that exposure with the one-vertical-wire method is good enough to allow hysterectomy, oophorectomy, adnexectomy, and treatment for ectopic pregnancy and endometriosis.

Other Procedures

Nephrectomy with SCLS for a small (less than 5 cm) renal-cell carcinoma has been reported by Nishimura and associates of Niigata, Japan.[10] They have

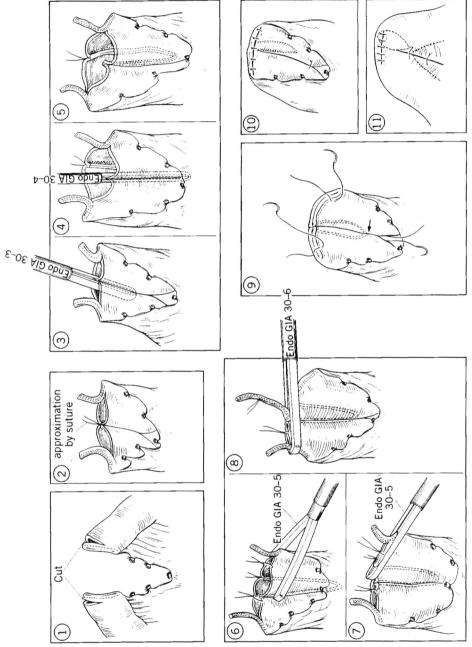

Figure 7.28. Intracorporeal reconstruction of the the the small intestine using a functional end-to-end

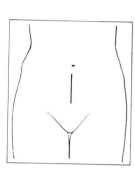

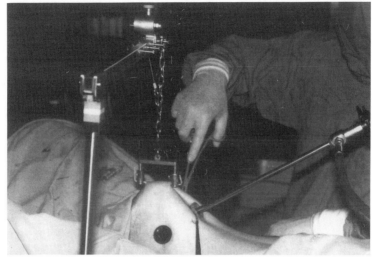

Figure 7.29 The subcutaneous lift system for gynecologic surgery designed by Isaka et al. Courtesy of Dr. K. Isaka.

added a 5-cm incision at the beginning of the operation and then applied SCLS for exposure of the kidney and surrounding tissues.[10] Miura and his colleagues of Niigata and Yamanaka and associates of Hyogo, Japan, have successfully performed hepatic resection with SCLS for a hepatocellular carcinoma. [10,11] Tamiya of Niigata has used the technique for splenectomy.[10] The authors have occasionally performed fenestration of liver cysts, partial resection of the stomach, and splenectomy.

V. PROBLEMS ENCOUNTERED WITH SCLS

Despite the technical and economical advantages of SCLS (because conventional instruments can be used), we must admit that many surgeons, even in Japan, feel uneasy about its usefulness in obese patients. We have encountered difficulties in our initial experience. In our early series we had several cases of poor exposure that led to either a combination of SCLS and insufflation or complete conversion to insufflation. However, we have improved the system extensively since the first trials and now believe that almost all Japanese patients with gallstones, except for rare cases of morbid obesity, can be treated with SCLS.

Key points for management of obese patients include:

1. Use as long a wire as possible.

2. Increase the number of wire-handle lifting sets to transform the abdominal wall into a kind of chest wall, or "costalization."

3. Raise the lifting sets to the maximum height. The skin withstands it well.

If these steps are carried out, a good view of the operative field should occur. Tables 7.3 and 7.4 show the relationship between obesity rate and view of the operative field in laparoscopic surgery with SCLS. Table 7.3 indicates the data one year before the modification and Table 7.4 during the recent 6 months. [Obesity rate is calculated as follows: (actual weight/standard weight-1)$\times$ 100; standard weight (kg) = height^2 (m^2)$\times$ 22).] The reader can see the remarkable progress made within two years.

The average rate of obesity of Japanese may be different from that of Americans and Europeans. Therefore, there is the possibility that our results may not be extrapolated to Western patients.

Smith and his colleagues recently published a textbook on a full-thickness wall lift entitled *Gasless Laparoscopy with Conventional Instruments: The*

TABLE 7.3

Relation between obesity rate and view of the field in the earlier series

Obesity rate (%)	No.	Poor view	(Insufflation)
$-20\sim$	2	0	
$-10\sim$	1	0	
$0\sim$	16	0	
$+10\sim$	15	0	
$+20\sim$	5	1	(0)
$+30\sim$	7	1	(0)
$+40\sim$	2	0	
$+50\sim$	1	0	
$+60\sim$	0		
$+70\sim$	1	1	(1)
Total	50	3	(1)

TABLE 7.4
Relation between obesity rate and view of the field in the recent series

Obesity rate (%)	No.	Poor view (insufflation)
–20~	1	0
–10~	9	0
0~	6	0
+ 10~	13	0
+20~	14	0
+30~	7	0
+40~	1	0
+50~	2*	0
+60~	1**	0
+70~	0	0
Total	54	0

*48 female (162 cm, 87 kg = 50%); 40 female (158 cm, 54 kg = 54%).
**39 female (148 cm, 78 kg = 62%).

Next Phase in Minimally Invasive Surgery.[8] They utilize a planar-lift retractor and report that the "exposure was generally adequate but was marginal in two morbidly obese patients in this series [of 32 attempts of gasless laparoscopic cholecystectomy]."[8a] Although our own experience with this planar-lift system is limited, we feel that better exposure can be obtained with SCLS. Hence the conclusion that SCLS might succeed in treating most American patients. More experience and objective studies are necessary for further evaluation.

VI. CONCLUSION, WITH A FUTURE PERSPECTIVE

The subcutaneous lift system is still being perfected and therefore is not yet in a form that allows for versatile use. Considering the high incidence of gastric cancer and the rapidly increasing number of colon cancers in Japan, laparoscopic or laparoscope-assisted surgery might well improve the quality of life of many more patients, if the procedure could become more refined so as to be safely applied to such cancer surgery. In this sense, the abdominal-wall lift holds great promise.

There is another reason for further development of abdominal-wall lift systems including SCLS. Wexner and associates have recently emphasized from an oncological viewpoint the risks associated with laparoscopic resection of colon cancer.[12] Besides cardiopulmonary and metabolic complications, CO_2 gas insufflation might incur adverse effects and enhance the chance of metastasis and invasion due to high sustained intraperitoneal pressure. If their concerns have a sound basis, the abdominal-wall lift should therefore replace gas insufflation in cancer surgery.

REFERENCES

1. Nagai H, Kondo Y, Yasuda T, et al.: "An abdominal wall-lift method of laparoscopic cholecystectomy without peritoneal insufflation." Surg Laparosc Endosc 1993, 3:175–179.

2. Smith RS, Fry WR, Tsoi EKM, et al.: "Gasless laparoscopy with conventional instruments: the next phase of minimally invasive surgery." Arch Surg 1993, 128:1102–1107.

3. Newman L, Luke JP, Ruben DM, et al.: "Laparoscopic herniorrhaphy without pneumoperitoneum." Surg Laparosc Endosc 1993, 3:213–215.

4. Hashimoto D, Nayeem SA, Kajiwara S, et al.: "Laparoscopic cholecystectomy: an approach without pneumoperitoneum." Surg Endosc 1993, 7:54–56.

5. Nagai H, Inaba T, Kamiya S, et al.: "A new method of laparoscopic cholecystectomy: An abdominal wall lifting technique without pneumoperitoneum." Surg Laparosc Endosc 1991, 1:126.

6. Mouret P, Francois Y: "Suspenseur de paroi et coelio-chirurgie." J Chir (Paris) 1992, 129:492–493.

7. Gazayerli MM: "The Gazayerli endoscopic retractor model 1." Surg Laparosc Endosc 1991, 1:98–100.

8. Smith RS, Organ CH Jr. (eds.), Gasless laparoscopy with conventional instruments: The next phase in minimaly invasive surgery. San Francisco: Norman Publishing, 1993.

8a. Henderson VJ, Tsoi EKM: "Gasless laparoscopy and biliary surgery." In Smith RS and Organ CH (eds.) Gasless Laparoscopy with Conventional Instruments: The Next Phase in Minimally Invasive Surgery. San Francisco: Norman Publishing 1993, 33–51.

9. 89th Congress of Kanto Area of Japanese Association of Obstetrics and Gynecology. June 11, 1995, Tokyo, Japan.

10. 5th Meeting of Niigata Endoscopic Surgery. January 21, 1975, Niigata, Japan.

11. Yamanaka N, Okamoto E, Tanaka T, et al.: "Techniques of laparoscopic hepatectomy." *Shujutsu,* 1995, 49:341–344.(in Japanese)

12. Wexner SD, Cohen SM: "Laparoscopic colectomy for malignancy: Advantages and limitations." Surg Oncol Clin North Am 1994, 3:637–643.

8

PLANAR LIFTING IN LAPAROSCOPIC SURGERY

Albert K. Chin, M.D.
Frederic H. Moll, M.D.

I. INTRODUCTION

Planar lifting refers to an abdominal-wall displacement concept developed to perform laparoscopic surgery without pneumoperitoneum. The technique of planar lifting was designed to allow the use of shorter, more conventional surgical instruments during laparoscopic procedures, and to permit the application of local or spinal anesthesia during these procedures. The abdominal wall assumes a domed configuration under traditional gas insufflation, leading to increased distances between peritoneal structures and the surface of the patient. The resultant elongation in instrument length limits dexterity during surgical manipulation and increases the learning curve associated with adoption of new laparoscopic procedures. Planar lifting generates an abdominal cavity characterized by a flat ceiling and provides adequate working space while avoiding excess abdominal displacement encountered with the dome of pneumoperitoneum.

Abdominal Access in Open and Laparoscopic Surgery
Edited by Edmund K. M. Tsoi and Claude H. Organ, Jr.
ISBN 0-471-13352-3 Copyright © 1966 by Wiley-Liss, Inc.

II. DEVELOPMENTAL HISTORY

Development of a method for mechanical displacement of the abdominal wall was initiated via experimentation with various techniques for achieving lift. The first attempt utilized a trocar sleeve with a distal-anchor balloon. Trocar insertion was followed by inflation of the balloon and suspension of the anchored sleeve to provide a source of abdominal lift. However, upon laparoscopic examination of the peritoneal cavity, it was found that this technique created only minimal working space, even though the abdominal wall was elevated a distance of 8–10 cm. Pliability of the abdomen led to tenting of the ventral wall, with limited expansion of the internal cavity.

Failure of single-point abdominal lift to provide a working laparoscopic field led to a study of linear lifting systems. Both wire cable and round rods were used to suspend the abdominal wall. The wire cable was approximately 3 mm in diameter. The rods were approximately 6 mm in diameter, and constructed of rigid metal and flexible nylon or fiberglass. A single wire cable or rod was passed in a transverse fashion, entering through an incision on one side of the abdomen and exiting through an incision on the opposite side. The rod was raised up on supports clamped to the side rail of the operating table, while the cable was raised on supports and further tightened using a winch system. A third incision was placed several centimeters inferior to the lifting rod or wire cable through which the laparoscope was introduced.

Examination of the space created by a linear-lifting method revealed that a rigid rod was superior to both a flexible rod and a wire cable in its ability to displace the abdominal wall. However, the maximal amount of working cavity available with linear lifting was restricted to a transverse section centered about the length of the lifting rod. The limited intraabdominal cavity formed by linear lifting hampered instrument insertion and surgical manipulation. The exposure afforded by a single line of lift was insufficient for general laparoscopic applications.

Failure of a linear-lifting system to provide adequate abdominal-wall retraction for widespread laparoscopic indications led to the realization that a planar system of lift was required for reliable working-cavity formation. Lifting structures were developed that resulted in planar abdominal displacement and incorporated the ability for insertion via a small incision. One early version involved a circular wire form, 15 cm in diameter, with a central vertical

stem for connection to a mechanical lifting arm. The wire structure was thread-
ed into the abdomen in a circumferential fashion via a 10-mm incision and lifted using a powered arm. Adequate abdominal-wall retraction was obtained
using this scheme; however, the circular-wire form resulted in a high incidence
of bowel and omental entrapment during placement. Its circumferential advancement technique gathered in surrounding tissue and bowel, similar to the
method in which a scythe gathers in wheat. The incorporated tissue had to be
removed prior to elevation of the abdominal wall.

An alternate version of a planar-lifting device was developed, based on
the geometric principle that two lines define a plane. This version involves a
fan retractor (Laparofan®, Origin Medsystems, Inc., Menlo Park, CA) that allows introduction through a 12-mm incision with the two legs of the fan in a
closed position. Upon fan deployment, the retractor creates a triangular plane
that is used to lift the abdomen (Figure 8.1) The fan retractor produces a laparoscopic cavity comparable to circular-wire form retraction, with the added
benefit of uncomplicated insertion and removal. Advancement of the fan retractor through an entry incision occurs in a linear fashion, and, if the abdominal wall is lifted slightly during fan insertion, there is decreased tendency for
extraneous tissue to be trapped by the fan blades.

Initial application of the fan retractor for abdominal-wall lifting by Tsoi
and Smith demonstrated the ability of the system to achieve successful laparoscopic cavity formation.[1] A small fraction of patients in this series suffered

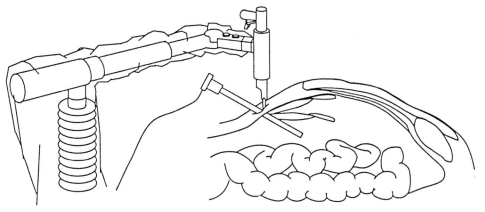

Figure 8.1. The fan retractor for planar lifting contains two legs that open up to form
a triangular lifting plane. The retractor attaches to a powered mechanical arm for abdominal-wall displacement.

from postoperative abdominal-wall tenderness. This pain was due to concentration of lifting force in the small surface area of the fan blades. The first fan blades were constructed of stainless steel rod approximately 5 mm in diameter. The rigidity of the blades, coupled with the tendency of the blade ends to poke into the abdominal wall upon retractor elevation, led to the occurrence of postoperative abdominal pain. Specialized fan blades were developed to produce an atraumatic means of lift. These blades contain stainless steel rods that extend halfway down the length of propeller-shaped plastic paddles. The propeller profile causes the proximal portion of the paddle to exhibit increased rigidity compared with the flattened distal end of the paddle, which is less rigid. Upon abdominal lifting, the modified fan blade flexes and assumes a curved configuration, mimicking the curvature of the abdominal wall under gas insufflation. Unlike the stainless steel rods, the wide, flattened tips of the fan retractor do not protrude into the abdominal wall. The composite metal and plastic fan retractor allows the application of planar lifting for extended laparoscopic procedures without concern for abdominal-wall trauma.

Elevation of the fan retractor is accomplished by a powered mechanical arm that attaches to the side rail of the operating table and connects to the retractor via a dovetail fitting. An electric-powered screw actuator located in the stem of the device provides vertical lift; a telescoping arm imparts reach in the horizontal plane. The perpendicular arrangement of tubular vertical and horizontal sections minimizes the profile of the lifting arm, resulting in an unobtrusive structure. Two separate pushbuttons control the elevation and descent of the lifting arm, thus maintaining simplicity of the lifting function.

The powered lifting arm contains a force limiter in its motor drive to reduce the potential for abdominal overdistention. The surface area of the anterior abdominal wall of an average-size adult was calculated using anthropometric data. Multiplication of the surface area by a pressure of 15 mm Hg yielded an equivalent vertical point force of 18 kg. The vertical drive of the powered arm is regulated so that the motor will stall at approximately 18 kg of lift. A separate manual hand crank lowers the arm in the event of electrical failure or allows lift above the 18-kg limit in procedures involving significant patient obesity. The fan retractor has a built-in spring gauge that indicates vertical force and provides additional feedback regarding the amount of applied lift.

III. OTHER PLANAR-LIFTING SYSTEMS

Two additional planar-lifting systems are being applied in laparoscopy.

Nagai described a multiple-wire system, which combines two or three linear lifting sources to create a functional plane of displacement (Figure 8.2).[2] Each lifting wire is introduced through the abdominal wall via entrance and exit incisions. An arrangement involving hoisting chains and a winching device suspends the assembly to produce abdominal lift. Widespread application of this technique has not occurred due to the various incisions and multiple steps required for system insertion.

François and Mouret describe a bent-wire form that is inserted through an abdominal incision and suspended by chain to maintain a laparoscopic working cavity (Figure 8.3).[3] This system employs a simpler insertion approach, compared with the multiple-wire approach just described. However, its utilization of a circumferential wire lifting form requires care upon peritoneal placement in order to avoid entrapment of bowel and omentum as the wire is guided into position.

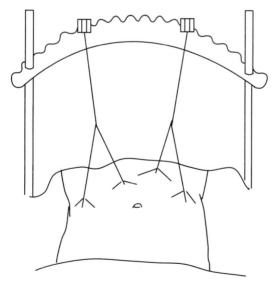

Figure 8.2. A multiple-wire system lifts the abdominal wall at various sites to yield a functional plane of displacement. The lifting wires can be suspended from a framework above the patient.

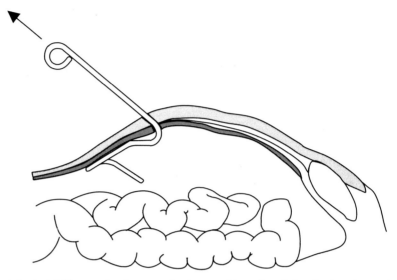

Figure 8.3. A rigid bent-wire form can be inserted into the abdominal cavity and suspended by chain to produce a planar type of lift.

IV. TECHNIQUE

The fan retractor is typically inserted via a minilaparotomy incision in the umbilical region. A 12- to 14-mm vertical or transverse incision is made at or below the umbilicus. The incision is carried down through the subcutaneous fat, and the linea alba identified and incised as well. The peritoneum is grasped with forceps, elevated above the midline incision, and incised sharply. The surgeon inserts a gloved finger into the abdomen to check for the presence of abdominal adhesions. A small right-angle retractor is inserted into the incision and pulled up to allow the closed tips of the fan retractor to be advanced into the abdomen. The surgeon removes the right-angle retractor and inserts the fan retractor, taking care to maintain the retractor blades parallel to the surface of the abdomen. Following full insertion of the blades, the fan retractor is swept in an arc in both directions. If there is no resistance against the fan blades, this indicates that the retractor has not trapped bowel and that significant adhesions are not present in the retraction area. The winged tabs are depressed to open the fan blades and the wedge lock slid down into position to keep the blades in an open position when the retractor is lifted. The free end of the sterile-draped lifting arm is telescoped out to mate with the dovetail connector on the fan retractor and the control button depressed to partially elevate the abdominal wall. The laparoscope is advanced into the fan insertion site into the angle between the deployed fan blades in order that the surgeon can visualize both blades and verify correct fan placement. After inspecting the surrounding bowel or omentum to ensure that neither has been incorporated by the retractor blades, the surgeon elevates the arm to the desired amount of abdominal lift.

Ancillary instrument ports are placed as required for the laparoscopic procedure. Valveless rigid or flexible sleeves can be used or, in some cases, a simple stab incision in the abdominal wall. A sleeve is placed behind the fan retractor in the lifting incision to keep the laparoscope clean during insertion. Access sites that accommodate multiple instrument exchanges utilize a sleeve to ensure that the instrument tip does not become caught on the peritoneum, which tends to peel away from the preperitoneal tissue. A slightly enlarged incision allows insertion of a gloved finger into the abdominal cavity for direct palpation, should this become necessary, or bowel can be exteriorized via such an incision for extraperitoneal surgery. Partially lowering the lifting arm achieves closer surgical access to intraabdominal organs. The planar ceiling permits endoscopic visualization without the risk of losing the dome effect that occurs with pneumoperitoneum. The improved access associated with planar lifting facilitates laparoscopic suturing, which may be performed with the use of conventional long-handled needle holders.

Fan-retractor positioning generally involves an umbilical entry site with a cephalad orientation of the retractor blades for upper abdominal procedures and a caudad orientation of the blades for lower abdominal and pelvic procedures. The lifting arm is secured to the side of the operating table opposite the primary surgeon. For upper abdominal procedures, the arm is placed at the level of the patient's shoulder. For lower abdominal pelvic work, the arm can be placed either at the level of the iliac crest or at shoulder level, depending upon the position of the surgical assistant and the placement of instrument ports. If the instrument handles extend toward the upper abdomen, the mechanical lifter is placed at the patient's hip to keep the superior portion of the abdominal field free from obstruction by the telescoping portion of the lifting arm.

Correct patient positioning is necessary to achieve proper surgical exposure in planar lifting. With mechanical abdominal-wall lifting, the absence of pneumoperitoneum results in more prominent bowel distention. To compensate for the lack of positive intraabdominal pressure that occurs with the planar-lifting technique and restricts the caliber of the bowel, the patient is tilted at an increased angle. For right upper quadrant procedures, the patient is placed in steep reversed Trendelenburg and turned towards the left side. For pelvic procedures, the patient is positioned in 30° or more of Trendelenburg. In addition, if necessary, a bowel retractor can be used to displace the bowel from the surgical site and to compress any remaining loops of bowel.

V. CLINICAL APPLICATIONS

Various laparoscopic procedures are being performed with the planar lifting technique. These procedures and the advantages gained by using the planar approach are as follows.

Cholecystectomy

For cholecystectomy, the 15-cm fan retractor can be introduced at the umbilicus and the fan blades directed toward the head of the patient. If the patient is obese, introduction of the fan retractor at a site midway between the umbilicus and the xiphoid can provide increased lift over the liver edge. As previously discussed, the patient is placed in reversed Trendelenburg and rolled toward the left side. If distended loops of bowel remain in the region of the gallbladder infundibulum, a laparoscopic grasper or blunt probe can be inserted adjacent to the endoscope at the fan insertion site to provide point retraction as needed. Planar lifting allows insertion of conventional instruments such as right-angle clamps to assist with dissection of the gallbladder and its vascular pedicle (Figure 8.4). This technique also allows continuous suction for evacuating smoke generated during electrosurgical application. If common bile duct exploration is indicated, the absence of gas-sealing ports facilitates the introduction and manipulation of balloon catheters and stone baskets.

Colectomy

In this procedure, the fan retractor is introduced via an umbilical incision. The fan blades are directed toward the pelvis for right and left hemicolectomy, sig-

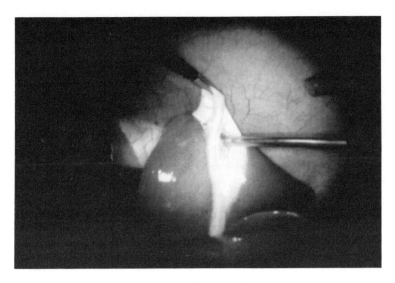

Figure 8.4. Cholecystectomy with planar lifting allows conventional instruments, such as Babcock clamps demonstrated here, to be used during laparoscopic dissection. (See insert for color representation.)

moid colectomy, and abdominoperineal resection. For transverse colectomy, the fan blades are deployed cephalad. In hemicolectomy, a 3-cm muscle-splitting incision for removing the specimen is placed in the lower quadrant on the side of the resection and a 10-mm ancillary instrument port is placed in the midline, midway between the umbilicus and the pubic symphysis. In transverse colectomy, the specimen-removal incision is created in the midline of the upper abdomen and two additional 10-mm working ports are placed on both sides at the mid-abdominal region. The specimen-removal site and the ancillary working ports allow simultaneous insertion of multiple instruments for retraction and manipulation. This capability for multiple instrument use via a single incision decreases the required number of access ports, compared with laparoscopic colectomy under gas insufflation, which requires multiple ports. The specimen-removal site allows the introduction of standard, nonlaparoscopic GIA staplers into the peritoneal cavity, substantially reducing the cost of the procedure. Exteriorization of the bowel via the 3-cm incision facilitates excision and reanastomosis. For tumor localization and lymph node evaluation, palpation can also be accomplished through the specimen-removal site. Suture ligation of omental vessels can be performed as well: planar lifting allows the index finger to be advanced through the abdominal wall for direct tensioning of extracorporeally formed knots, eliminating the need for knot-pushing devices. Upon completion of the anastomosis, planar lifting permits identification of residual bleeding sites that might otherwise be masked under positive-pressure conditions existent with pneumoperitoneum.

Laparoscopic-Assisted Vaginal Hysterectomy

Planar lifting is particularly useful for maintaining endoscopic visualization in laparoscopic-assisted vaginal hysterectomy (Figure 8.5). Pelvic orientation of the 10-cm fan retractor is typically used, with the patient placed in significant Trendelenburg position to permit the bowel to recede from the operative site. Devascularization of the uterus and detachment of suspensory uterine ligaments can be performed with the use of conventional open surgical instruments inserted via bilateral abdominal-access incisions. Upon completion of the abdominal portion of uterine mobilization, subsequent dissection is conducted from a vaginal approach. With planar lifting, no loss of laparoscopic visualization occurs when the vaginal cuff is incised because no pneumoperitoneum is present to deflate. Mechanical abdominal retraction allows simultaneous inspection of the operative site from an intraabdominal vantage point as well as from a transvaginal approach.

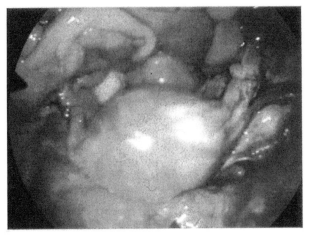

Figure 8.5. A view of the uterus during laparoscopic-assisted vaginal hysterectomy utilizing planar lifting. (See insert for color representation.)

Aortoiliac Reconstruction

Laparoscopic aortobifemoral and iliofemoral bypass procedures have also been performed using planar abdominal-wall lifting.[4] The ability to conduct endoscopic procedures without the use of gas insufflation is critical to aortic surgery for several reasons. First, it minimizes the potential for sudden interruption of laparoscopic visualization due to deflation of the pneumoperitoneum. Collapse of the working field during a critical juncture in the aortic anastomosis could result in the loss of vascular control. Second, planar abdominal-wall lifting eliminates the concerns regarding the occurrence of gas embolism in the event of injury to the great vessels. Third, the ability to use conventional surgical instrumentation, including vascular needle holders, simplifies the placement of vascular clamps and the application of anastomotic sutures. Aortoiliac reconstruction via a transabdominal laparoscopic approach proceeds with the placement of a periumbilical fan retractor oriented towards the pelvis. A 3-cm muscle-splitting incision is performed in the left lower quadrant. This incision is used for the introduction of multiple laparotomy pads used in bowel packing, various instruments for aortic dissection and bowel retraction, and needle holders for completion of the proximal anastomosis. Considerable effort may be required to achieve sufficient bowel retraction for initial aortic isolation. The operating table is rolled towards the patient's right side and multiple laparotomy pads are applied to sequester the bowel from the aortic area. Following successful aortic exposure, placement of the graft proceeds. Aortic crossclamps can be applied via ancillary-access incisions. The proximal anastomosis is performed through the minilaparotomy incision, with visualization provided by laparoscopic imaging and direct viewing via the 3-cm incision. Planar lifting allows the surgeon to perform this major vascular procedure using a minimum amount of incisions.

Preperitoneal Applications

A group of preperitoneal laparoscopic procedures has been developed. These procedures involve formation of a total extraperitoneal working cavity using balloon-assisted dissection and maintenance of the cavity through gas insufflation or planar lifting.[5-7] Total preperitoneal procedures allow laparoscopic procedures to be performed without entry into the peritoneal cavity, thus avoiding potential postoperative adhesion formation. These procedures also provide an opportunity for laparoscopic procedures to be performed under local or regional anesthesia. Because intraabdominal gas insufflation is not utilized, CO_2-induced peritoneal discomfort is absent and mechanical ventilation is not required. Application of planar lifting to preperitoneal surgery extends the benefits of conventional instrument use and simplified suturing technique to these procedures. Preperitoneal laparoscopic procedures that make use of planar lifting include the following:

Inguinal Hernia Repair. A 12-mm infraumbilical incision is made through the skin and dissection is carried out at the medial border of the rectus muscle. The anterior rectus sheath is incised, the rectus muscle displaced bluntly, and the posterior rectus sheath identified. A balloon dissection cannula (PDB® Cannula, Origin Medsystems, Inc., Menlo Park, CA) is advanced to the pubic symphysis via this incision, the laparoscope placed within the balloon, and the balloon inflated with a squeeze bulb to form a preperitoneal cavity under direct vision (Figure 8.6). The dissection balloon is deflated and removed, and a 10-cm fan retractor is introduced into the incision. The fan retractor is directed towards the pelvis, opened, and elevated to support the ceiling of the preperitoneal cavity. A 5-mm probe is introduced via the fan insertion incision to displace the peritoneum downward and expand the cavity in preparation for instrument-port placement. The laparoscope is inserted in the same incision. Dissection of the cord structures, reduction of the hernia sac, and placement of prosthetic mesh are all conducted in the preperitoneal cavity.

Bladder Neck Suspension. Extraperitoneal Burch procedures can be approached as described above by balloon preparation of the preperitoneal space followed by planar lifting of the laparoscopic working cavity. Bilateral suture placement in paraurethral vaginal tissue and suspension from Cooper's ligament are facilitated by the use of a gasless technique. Possible routine use of spinal anesthesia during this procedure is a benefit of the total extraperitoneal approach.

Lymphadenectomy. Lymph-node sampling for cancer staging is easily accomplished in the preperitoneal space. Midline inflation of the balloon dissection cannula allows access for bilateral lymph-node resection. An infraumbilical incision is used, as in the preperitoneal procedures previously described. The limited surgical and anesthetic morbidity associated with the total

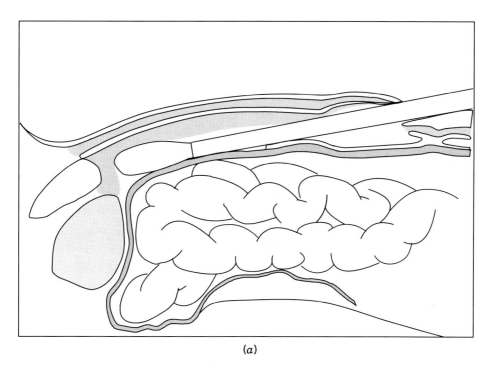

(a)

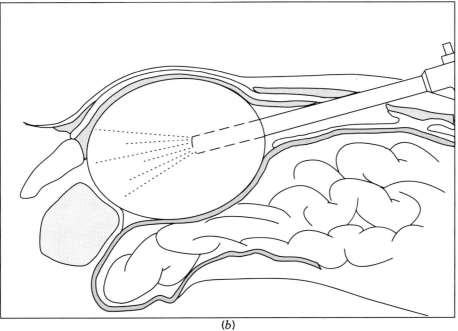

(b)

Figure 8.6. The balloon dissection cannula for extraperitoneal dissection. (a) The cannula is advanced to the symphysis pubis. (b) With the laparoscope placed inside the cannula, the balloon is inflated under direct vision to form a cavity in the pre-peritoneal space.

preperitoneal approach makes this procedure attractive for elderly patients with prostatic or pelvic malignancies.

Balloon dissection of the preperitoneal space for bladder-neck suspension and lymphadenectomy generally involves the use of a spherical, elastomeric balloon cannula. Midline advancement and inflation of the balloon cannula results in a centrally located one-liter cavity with good access to the space of Retzius. During inflation, the laparoscope resides within the balloon and provides visual assurance of correct cannula placement through the transparent balloon membrane. Appearance of a yellow color on the laparoscopic picture indicates correct balloon position within the preperitoneal fat layer. Inadvertent advancement of the cannula into the rectus muscle is observed as red coloration outside the balloon, while passage of the cannula through the peritoneum into the abdominal cavity is appreciated by visualization of bowel through the laparoscope. Upon balloon inflation, preperitoneal landmarks come into view. The curved, white arch of Cooper's ligament tends to be the most prominent landmark. The epigastric vessels may also be observed.

For bilateral inguinal hernia repair, preparation of the preperitoneal working cavity utilizes an alternate version of balloon dissection cannula. A relatively nonelastomeric, kidney-shaped balloon (Figure 8.7) is used to dissect a preperitoneal cavity that extends laterally to provide bilateral access to the internal inguinal ring. The ensheathed balloon unrolls in opposite directions from the midline cannula position to form the desired working space. The lap-

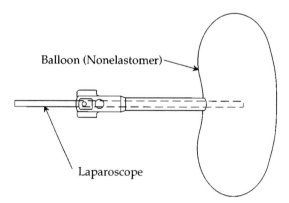

Balloon (Nonelastomer)

Laparoscope

Figure 8.7. A kidney-shaped balloon is used for bilateral hernia repair. The balloon is initially ensheathed then unrolls upon inflation to form a cavity with bilateral extensions in the preperitoneal space.

aroscope is also placed within this balloon to permit observation of the dissection process.

Retroperitoneal Applications

An approach similar to that described for preperitoneal applications, namely, balloon dissection of a working cavity and planar support of the dissected space, can also be applied to the retroperitoneal region. Initial entry is gained by a 14-mm left-flank incision. Fibers of the external oblique and transversus abdominis muscles are bluntly separated and finger dissection through the perinephric fat clears a path to the infrarenal space. A balloon dissection cannula is advanced through this tract and inflated to expose the left kidney, the left adrenal gland, the ureter, the aorta, the periaortic lymph nodes, and the vena cava. A specialized longitudinal balloon cannula (Figure 8.8) can be substituted for the spherical balloon dissector and inflated to create an elongated cavity extending from the infrarenal aorta to the aortic bifurcation. The dissection balloon is deflated and removed prior to insertion of a 10-cm fan retractor, which is lifted by the mechanical arm to maintain the ceiling of the retroperitoneal cavity. An inflatable flat, elliptical balloon retractor is introduced via a separate 12-mm incision to displace the dissected peritoneum medially. Together, the planar lifting retractor and the elliptical balloon retractor are sufficient to support a retroperitoneal cavity for the duration of a laparoscopic procedure.

The retroperitoneal approach is useful for laparoscopic nephrectomy and adrenalectomy procedures. Infrarenal placement of the balloon dissector provides ready exposure of the renal vessels for control and ligation. Retroperi-

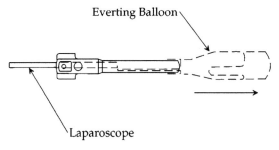

Figure 8.8. A specialized dissection cannula uses a balloon that is inverted into the cannula. The balloon everts upon inflation to dissect a longitudinal cavity.

toneal access also offers significant potential for reducing bowel retraction requirements in aortobifemoral bypass procedures. A single balloon retractor
can be used to displace the peritoneum and the abdominal contents medially,
an accomplishment normally achieved through the use of multiple bowel retractors and laparotomy pads during a transabdominal approach. Isolation of
the aorta allows periaortic lymphadenectomy to proceed through limited-ac-
cess incisions. Retraction of the aorta and vena cava clears a path to the spine;
this approach provides a means for retroperitoneal laparoscopic discectomy
and spinal fusion. As outlined in the case of aortic reconstruction, a retroperitoneal mechanical-lift technique is particularly useful for achieving laparoscopic spinal access without the necessity of dealing with substantial bowel retraction.

VI. ANCILLARY INSTRUMENTS IN PLANAR LIFTING

Bowel Retractors

Adequate bowel retraction is essential for successful exposure in laparoscopic
planar-lift procedures. The use of multifingered, flat-bladed fan retractors is
helpful when retraction of one or two loops of bowel is required at a specific
site. If widespread bowel retraction is needed, a means of applying pressure
over a broad surface area is utilized. A broad, continuous retraction surface can
be provided by an elliptical balloon retractor, which is composed of a flat, inflatable retractor connected to a long shaft that also serves as the balloon inflation lumen. The elliptical balloon retractor is designed to incorporate a high
degree of flexural and torsional rigidity while maintaining a smooth tissue-
contact interface. Multibladed retractors contain gaps between the blades,
which allow bowel to squeeze through upon downward retractor pressure.
The continuous surface of the balloon retractor acts to wall off an operating
site against bowel encroachment. Two versions of the inflatable retractor can
be applied (Figure 8.9). The first version employs an inflation shaft that lies in
the same plane with the flat elliptical balloon. This version is used to exert simple downward pressure on the bowel or retracted organ. The second version
consists of an elliptical balloon that is oriented perpendicular to the inflation
shaft. This configuration allows the balloon retractor to be applied as a rake,
gathering in bowel and holding it away from the surgical site.

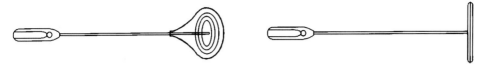

Figure 8.9. Elliptical balloon retractors. The first version (left) uses a balloon in the same plane as the inflation shaft; the second version (right) uses a balloon placed perpendicular to the inflation shaft to allow the retractor to gather in and retain the bowel.

If retraction requirements in generalized bowel distention exceed the ability of handheld retractors to maintain control, multiple conventional surgical laparotomy sponges can be inserted via a small abdominal incision. Moistened sponges can be deployed over exposed bowel surfaces to weigh down and confine the movable bowel mass. The laparotomy pads produce an effect similar to gas insufflation and also control bowel expansion as the laparoscopic case progresses.

Access Ports

Gas-sealing trocar sleeves are not required in planar lifting because mechanical retractors maintain the endoscopic cavity. This increases the simplicity of laparoscopic procedures and changes the technique of access-port creation. Rigid and flexible valveless sleeves can be inserted through abdominal incision sites to maintain access for instrument insertion. A sharpened obturator can be used to facilitate access port advancement; however, a deep or full-thickness incision of adequate length should be made prior to sleeve placement. With planar lifting, no pneumoperitoneum is present to provide back support against trocar placement. To guard against inadvertant overloading of the fan retractor blades, a deep incision is created at port placement sites.

Flexible ports permit the insertion of curved instruments such as Metzenbaum scissors or right-angle clamps. Use of conventional hinged instruments is further enhanced if the flexible port is slit along its entire length. The slitted port functions as a small, full-thickness abdominal incision, with little restriction on the opening and closing of instruments about their pivot point. Unlike a simple abdominal incision, however, the slitted port provides unimpeded transabdominal access and prevents potential instrument entrapment in the preperitoneal space.

Specialized Instruments

Planar-lift procedures permit the use of longer versions of conventional surgical instruments such as vascular instruments and retractors. The additional length allows surgical access from instrument ports that are somewhat removed from the operative site. Straight, curved, and right-angle clamps, Babcock clamps, and long needle holders are all useful for performing planar-lift laparoscopic procedures. The familiarity that surgeons possess with instruments used during open surgery makes their use more attractive in the endoscopic setting. Traditional ring handles and pivot jaws incorporated in these instruments confer greater control during surgical manipulation when compared with laparoscopic versions, which have long shafts and short working jaws.

Limitations of conventional surgical instruments in planar lifting are associated with interactions between the abdominal wall and instrument pivot points in patients of variable obesity. Although pliable, a thick abdominal wall restricts the ability of instrument handles to open. The pivot point could be modified to address this limitation. Alternatively, instruments are being developed with different linkage schemes to permit activation of the working end while limiting the width of the handle during device actuation.

VII. LIMITATIONS OF FAN RETRACTION FOR PLANAR LIFTING

The fan retractor functions well in the majority of laparoscopic applications. However, it provides a surgical cavity different from that provided by pneumoperitoneum. Mechanical abdominal lifting with the fan retractor results in a peritoneal cavity that contains a trapezoidal cross section, whereas gas insufflation results in an elliptical cross section (Figure 8.10). This difference leads to two changes in surgical exposure. First, the lateral margins of the cavity have a truncated appearance, rather than the rounded profile experienced with pneumoperitoneum. Visualization of the paracolic gutters is compromised bilaterally. Although visualization of this region may not be clinically important, the surgeon may sense confinement in the resultant working space. Second, the ceiling of the peritoneal cavity is flat rather than dome-shaped. However, due to the trapezoidal configuration obtained with fan-retractor lifting, a smaller

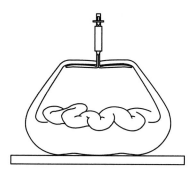 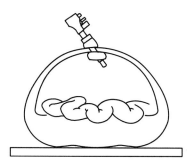

Figure 8.10. The trapezoidal configuration observed with the fan-retractor method of planar lifting (left) is contrasted with the elliptical cavity experienced upon gas insufflation (right).

laparoscopic cavity exists. Loss of vertical height within the cavity improves access to intraabdominal organs, but it may hamper performance of some procedures in obese patients.

Bowel distention resulting from the absence of positive pressure within the peritoneal cavity may further decrease the height of the laparoscopic space. In the majority of cases, bowel retraction at specific locations provides adequate control for successful visualization. If additional or more generalized retraction is required, moistened laparotomy sponges can be introduced via instrument-access incisions to blanket the bowel and decrease the amount of distention.

The limited surface-lifting area of the fan blades may lead to postoperative abdominal-wall discomfort following lengthy laparoscopic procedures; complaints of abdominal-wall tenderness usually do not occur until the operative time exceeds three hours. The incidence of muscle trauma incurred by the lifting blades is very rare. This is due to the distal flexibility of the blades, which allows them to assume a curved contour, thus ensuring that the tips do not project into muscle tissue upon planar lifting.

VIII. NEW DEVELOPMENTS IN PLANAR LIFTING

Further developments in planar lifting address the limitations noted in present fan retractors. Most notable of these involves the truncated working space and trapezoidal cavity observed with the lifting fan. An alternate technique that employs a circular inflatable disc as the lifting device has been developed (Figure 8.11). The balloon lift is inserted into the abdominal cavity through a 14-mm incision, inflated, and attached to the mechanical arm. An opening in the center of the balloon lift permits introduction of the laparoscope. The circular lifting disc is centered about the incision, directing lift towards both the upper abdomen and the pelvis, and providing support in the lateral reaches of the abdominal wall. Laparoscopic exposure is increased with this device, the wide circular lifting profile decreases the trapezoidal effect, and the expanded cavity allows bowel migration out of the surgical area. The contact area of the lifting balloon is much greater than the corresponding surface area of the fan retractor. This provides a gentler method of abdominal-wall suspension. The slippery face of the balloon lift makes it impossible to compress the bowel against the ventral surface of the abdominal wall. Trapped bowel loops slide off the balloon lift upon elevation by the mechanical arm.

Another area of focus in laparoscopic research involves the development of structural balloons. Planar lifting was developed to perform laparoscopic surgery through the use of an external lifting mechanism, thus eliminating the need for gas insufflation. An alternate method of achieving laparoscopic exposure without pneumoperitoneum involves the use of internal support structures. Internal balloon structures are a logical choice, as they enable a significant number of instruments to be introduced into the peritoneal cavity via small openings because the balloons deploy into large supporting frameworks upon inflation. Structural balloons are composed of two

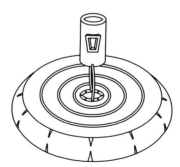

Figure 8.11. The balloon lifter consists of an inflatable disc that has a central hole for endoscope insertion. It is tethered to a connector that attaches to the mechanical lifting arm.

components: a large inner cavity that is inflated to displace the abdominal wall or dissect an extraperitoneal space, and an outer strut system that is inflated secondarily to maintain the space formed by the first balloon component (Figure 8.12). Incisions can be made through the first balloon, in regions not occupied by struts of the second inflatable component, to allow introduction of the laparoscope and surgical instruments. The first balloon or inner cavity is deflated upon incision; however, the laparoscopic cavity is supported by the inflated struts. This scheme retains the benefits of planar lifting in terms of conventional surgical instrument application, potential for local or regional anesthesia use, continuous smoke evacuation, and ability for limited palpation. The disadvantage is its limitation upon instrument placement,

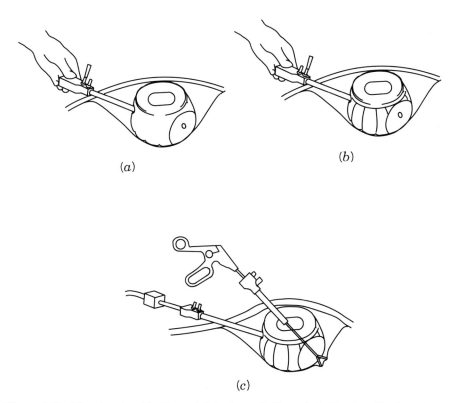

(a)

(b)

(c)

Figure 8.12. The structural balloon: (a) the inner balloon is inflated to displace tissue and form a working cavity; (b) the outer strut system is inflated to maintain the cavity; (c) windows between the inflated struts are incised to allow instrument passage and tissue access.

which must occur between strut locations, and its limitation upon operative-site access, which is dependent upon structural balloon orientation within the endoscopic cavity. Individualized balloon configurations with varying strut designs will enable specific procedures to be performed under structural balloon support.

IX. CONCLUSIONS

The development of a planar lifting laparoscopic technique has broadened the range of instrument use and altered the operative approach in minimally invasive surgery. The impact of this development is associated with its ability to bring more technically demanding procedures into the realm of endoscopic surgery. Its full potential is still to be appreciated, as research into additional gasless surgical techniques continues to be conducted. The results to date have been very encouraging, with observed improvements in surgical manipulation, anesthesia usage, and postoperative patient comfort. Planar lifting appears to be an approach that will go hand in hand with future innovative laparoscopic development. Its practicality will drive the progression to additional novel endoscopic applications. Combination of planar-lifting principles with other burgeoning technologies will perhaps result in future techniques whose advent will be appreciated by patient and surgeon alike.

REFERENCES

1. Tsoi EKM, Smith RS, Fry WR, et al.: "Laparoscopic surgery without pneumoperitoneum. A preliminary report." Surg Endosc 1994, 8:382–383.

2. Nagai H, Kondo Y, Yasuda T, et al.: "An abdominal wall-lift method of laparoscopic cholecystectomy without peritoneal insufflation." Surg Laparosc Endosc 1993, 3(3): 175–179.

3. François Y, Mouret P: "Suspenseur de paroi et coelio-chirurgie." J Chir (Paris) 1992, 129(11):492–493.

4. Berens ES, Herde JR: Laparoscopic aortofemoral and iliofemoral bypass. American College of Surgeons. 80th Annual Clinical Congress. Vascular Surgery Motion Picture Session, 1994.

5. Ferzli GS, Dysarz FA III: "Extraperitoneal endoscopic inguinal herniorrhaphy performed without carbon dioxide insufflation." J Laparoendosc Surg 1994, 4(5):301–304.

6. Albert P, Raboy A: "Extraperitoneal endoscopic node dissection—without gas." Contemp Urol 1994, March:50–56.

7. Chin AK, Moll FH, McColl MB: "Balloon-assisted extraperitoneal laparoscopic hernia repair." In Darzi A, Monson JRT (eds.), Laparoscopic Inguinal Hernia Repair (Oxford: Isis Medical Media, 1994), 70–90.

9

LAPAROSCOPIC PROCEDURES USING THE PLANAR-LIFTING TECHNIQUE

Edmund K. M. Tsoi, M.S., M.D.

I. INTRODUCTION

In Chapter 8, Chin and Moll described the development of the planar abdominal-wall lifter and its application. The initial investigation in experimental animals with the planar-lifting technique for gasless laparoscopic procedures showed great promise for its role in minimally invasive surgery. One of its main benefits is that it provides adequate exposure for laparoscopic procedures without causing cardiopulmonary side effects. A clinical trial conducted in 1992 at the University of California–Davis (UCD), East Bay Department of Surgery further reinforced the experimental findings and established the planar-lift method as the access and exposure technique of choice for a variety of laparoscopic cases.[1] This chapter will discuss the access technique of various

Abdominal Access in Open and Laparoscopic Surgery
Edited by Edmund K. M. Tsoi and Claude H. Organ, Jr.
ISBN 0-471-13352-3 Copyright © 1966 by Wiley-Liss, Inc.

gasless laparoscopic procedures performed with the planar abdominal-lifting device.

II. DIAGNOSTIC LAPAROSCOPY

The role of laparoscopy in evaluating and managing hemodynamically stable trauma patients has increased as surgeons become more comfortable with minimally invasive surgery. Critics of the minimally invasive technique are concerned about the potential cardiovascular problems associated with pneumoperitoneum as well as the inability to perform a complete small bowel exploration, inspect the retroperitoneum, and examine abdominal contents by palpation. The concern for tension pneumothorax during laparoscopy in patients with diaphragmatic laceration(s) makes planar lifting for exposure especially attractive. Limited digital and direct visual examination of intraabdominal contents are possible. In addition, the small bowel can easily be examined intracorporeally or extracorporeally via a miniincision. Inspection of the retroperitoneal structure is adequate but experience is required to master the technique of retroperitoneoscopy.

All hemodynamically stable patients with blunt or penetrating abdominal trauma are eligible for gasless laparoscopy. Since we are interested in performing both diagnostic and therapeutic laparoscopy, all laparoscopic procedures are performed in the operating room under general anesthesia. A designated equipment cart containing the necessary laparoscopic instruments is set aside in the operating room to permit rapid access to the instruments.

The electrical-powered Laparolift® (Origin Medsystems Inc., Menlo Park, CA) is mounted onto the siderail of the operating table before the patient is draped. A small (< 2 cm) periumbilical incision is made to enter the abdomen. The abdominal wall is lifted vertically with an Army–Navy retractor. A Laparofan® abdominal-wall retractor is carefully inserted into the abdomen under direct visualization. The fan blade is pointed at the upper abdomen first or in the direction of the suspected injured organ. The blade is carefully opened before it is connected to the sterilely draped telescopic arm of the Laparolift® (Figure 9.1). By activating a switch on the telescopic arm, the abdominal wall is elevated to a maximum pressure of 18 kg. A 0° or 30° laparoscope is placed into the abdomen via the same periumbilical incision made for the Laparofan®. Frequently, a 5-mm endoscopic grasper is placed into the same peri-

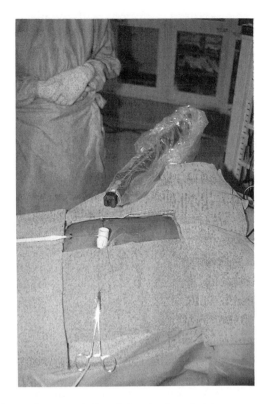

Figure 9.1. The telescopic arm of the abdominal wall lifter covered with a sterile drape is placed into the sterile field. (See insert for color representation.)

umbilical incision to manipulate abdominal contents. Two or more small incisions (< 1 cm) or trocars are placed at the lateral rectus border, and either in the mid-epigastric region or the suprapubic area for placement of additional endoscopic graspers or retractors (Figure 9.2). After examination of the upper abdomen or the suspected injured organ, the abdominal wall is lowered by activating another switch on the telescopic arm. The Laparofan® blade is closed and redirected to the pelvis or to another injured organ. Again, the blade is reopened, the abdominal wall is elevated, and laparoscopy continues.

In cases where the injured organ is identified (such as a laceration in the small bowel), the periumbilical incision is extended by 3–4 cm or a separate incision (< 5 cm) is made to exteriorize the injured bowel for repair. This new access can also be used for introducing conventional instruments to repair the organ intracorporeally (Figure 9.3a).

Gasless laparoscopy has also been used in nontrauma patients with a di-

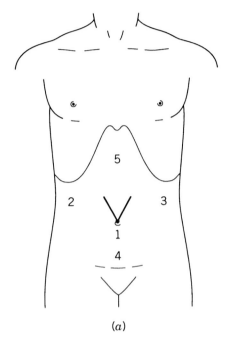

(a)

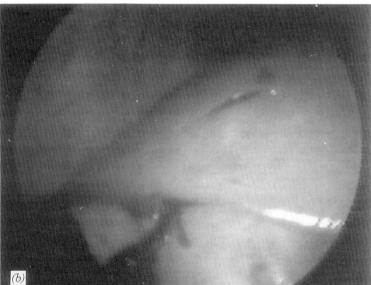

Figure 9.2. (a) Diamond-shaped access placement for diagnostic laparoscopy. Access number 5 can be omitted for limited pelvic peritoneoscopy. (b) Liver laceration caused by stabbing identified during trauma laparoscopy. (See insert for color representation.)

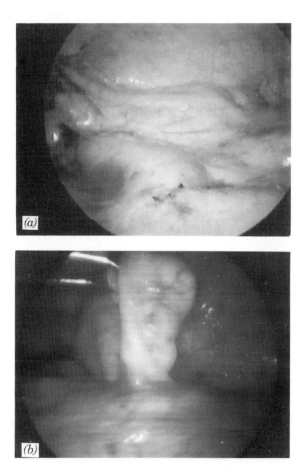

Figure 9.3. (a) Small bowel laceration was identified during diagnostic laparoscopy and placed back into the abdomen after repaired extracorporeally with silk sutures. (b) A normal appendix is being examined with the help of an Allis clamp. (See insert for color representation.)

agnosis of abdominal pain to rule out surgical disease. The patient usually has undergone ultrasound or other diagnostic radiographic studies prior to laparoscopy. Although continuous intravenous sedation together with local anesthesia may be used to perform diagnostic laparoscopy, most of the author's patients have undergone general anesthesia for comfort reasons.

The placement of the Laparofan®, small incisions, or trocars for surgical instruments in elective diagnostic laparoscopy is similar to that of trauma patients. In cases where diagnostic laparoscopy is used to rule out appendicitis (Figure 9.3b), the right paramedian incision or trocar is initially omitted until appendicitis is confirmed (Figure 9.4). It is because this author does not rou-

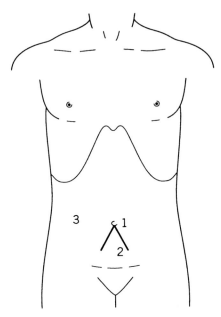

Figure 9.4. Diagram showing access placement for pelvic peritoneoscopy. Access 1 can be used for placement of the Laparofan®, laparoscope, and a 5-mm endoscopic grasper. Access 3 is placed cephalad to McBurney's point.

tinely perform incidental appendectomy; therefore, a scar in the right lower quadrant area can confuse other surgeon who may be examining the patient for possible appendicitis. Diagnostic laparoscopy may be employed for diagnostic purposes to rule out surgical disease in patients who have complex medical problems when physical examination, blood tests, radiography, and analysis of the patients' medical history have failed to rule out acute abdominal process (Figures 9.5 and 9.6). However, this author must caution the reader to use diagnostic laparoscopy only if one has considerable experience with this procedure or if another senior staff member is available to assist in identifying the pathology.

III. UPPER ABDOMINAL PROCEDURES

Cholestectomy

Laparoscopic cholecystectomy using the planar abdominal lifter can be accomplished with three or four accesses. A periumbilical incision is used for

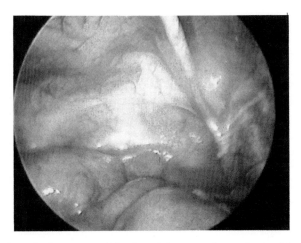

Figure 9.5. Purulent drainage noted in the abdomen of a patient with HIV disease and nonspecific abdominal pain. (See insert for color representation.)

placement of the abdominal-wall lifter; a right subcostal incision may be used instead if the patient had previous abdominal surgery. A 5-mm laparoscopic grasper is usually placed via the first access (behind the laparoscopic) to manipulate the gallbladder. This maneuver allows the surgeon to determine the laparoscopic operability of his or her case. The second access is placed at the subxiphoid area, just lateral to the fan blade or the recently introduced inflated Airlift® abdominal wall lifter (Figure 9.7). The third and if necessary the

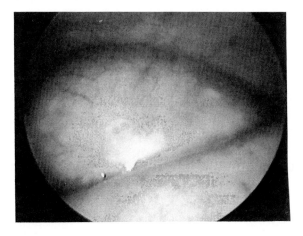

Figure 9.6. Ischemic cecum with purulent exudate noted during diagnostic laparoscopy. (See insert for color representation.)

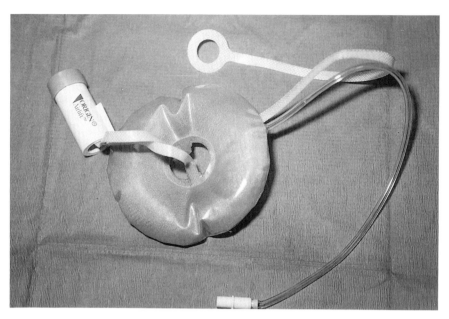

Figure 9.7. Picture of the inflatable abdominal wall lifter—Airlift®. (See insert for color representation.)

fourth accesses are in the right subcostal area, usually at a much more inferi-or position than those used for trocars in conventional laparoscopic cholecys-tectomy (Figures 9.8a and b). Cholangiography can be done by placing the cholangio-catheter via any one of the accesses without removing the abdom-inal-wall lifter but the radiopaque telescopic arm of the Laparolift® must be moved out of the x-ray field. Common bile duct exploration and choledocho-scope can be facilitated with a separate right paramedian miniincision. This access can also be used for instrument placement during the closure of the choledochus.

Gastric Procedures

Gasless laparoscopic gastrostomy can be done under local anesthesia with in-travenous sedation. The indications for laparoscopic placement of enteral ac-cess have been discussed in Chapter 4; these patients are not candidates for percutaneous enteral feeding access placement. The first access is placed in the supraumbilical position for insertion of the abdominal-wall lifter and the la-paroscope. The second access is placed at or just left of the midline in the sub-

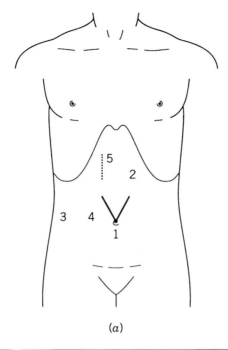

(a)

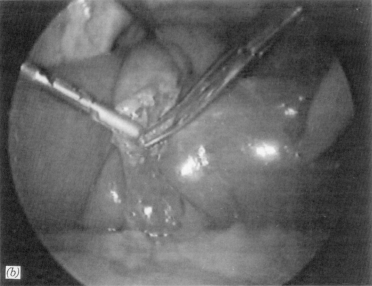

(b)

Figure 9.8. (a) Diagram showing access for laparoscopic cholecystectomy. Access 5 is a miniparamedian incision used for choledochoscopy and suturing of the choledochus. (b) Isolation of the cystic duct of an inflamed gallbladder using a tonsil clamp. (See insert for color representation.)

xiphoid area. The third access is placed halfway between the umbilicus and the left subcostal margin; this access is used for grasping the stomach with endoscopic graspers and for anchoring the gastrostomy tube as well as the stomach to the anterior abdominal wall (Figure 9.9). The author prefers to use an 18 French or bigger Foley catheter for laparoscopic gastrostomy.

Besides gastrostomy, similar access has also been used at UCD–East Bay to perform a modified version of Graham's patch as well as for closure of traumatic gastric perforation of the stomach. In the latter procedure, paramedian mini incisions are used for access to close the gastrostomy (Figure 9.10).[2]

The pros and cons of gasless laparoscopic surgery will be discussed in Chapter 10; one of the drawbacks that hinders the development of using the planar abdominal retractor for upper abdominal procedures is diaphragmatic movements causing respiratory variation in the position of intraabdominal structures. Because of such movements, the dissection of the esophageal hiatus is more difficult than when using CO_2 pneumoperitoneum for exposure. However, with the gasless technique, one can eliminate the concern of tension

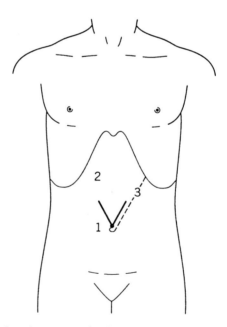

Figure 9.9. Diagram showing access for laparoscopic gastrostomy. The dotted line represents an imaginary line drawn from the umbilicus to the mid point of the left lower rib; access 3 is placed at the midpoint of this imaginary line for the gastrostomy.

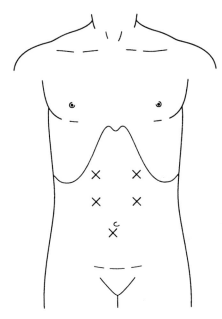

Figure 9.10. Diagram showing the access used in closure of traumatic gastric perforation.

pneumothorax associated with CO_2 insufflation. Using the planar-lifting technique, the author has successfully reduced the gastric volvulus and performed anterior gastropexy in a patient with a large hiatal hernia and complex medical problems (Figure 9.11). However, suboptimal exposure of the esophageal hiatus is noted in performing antireflux procedures.

Liver Biopsy

Laparoscopic liver biopsy is indicated for patients who have coagulopathy and in cases where diagnosis has failed after percutaneous biopsy. The first access is placed at the supraumbilical incision; the second and third access are placed in the right and left paramedian area (Figure 9.12). A conventional 5-mm trocar is used as one of the access because the trocar gas port can be used to evacuate the smoke generated by the electrocautery during dissection. Scissors with bipolar coagulating ability have been used for taking a generous wedge sample (Figure 9.13). Samples of the deep liver parenchyma can also be obtained with the conventional Tru-Cut™ biopsy needle.

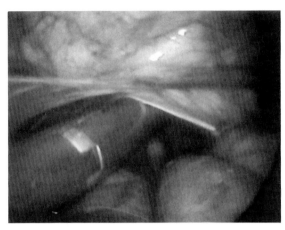

Figure 9.11. Gastric volvulus in the hiatal hernia is being reduced back into the abdomen with an endoscopic grasper. (See insert for color representation.)

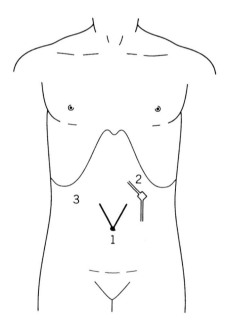

Figure 9.12. Diagram showing access for liver biopsy. Access 2 represents a conventional trocar connected to continuous suction to evacuate the smoke generated during cauterization.

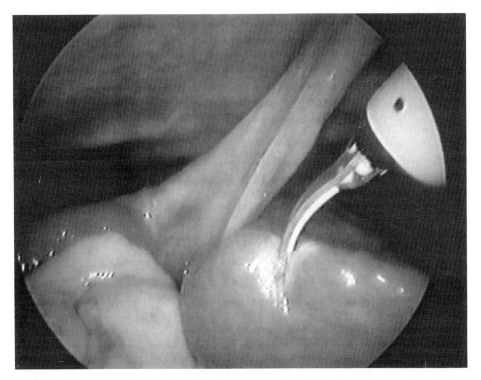

Figure 9.13. A small liver wedge is being removed with bipolar scissors. (See insert for color representation.)

III. COLON PROCEDURES

Colectomy

At UCD–East Bay, great skepticism exists concerning the value of laparoscopic colectomy in the treatment of malignant disease. Reports of tumor recurrence at the trocar sites make surgeons even less enthusiastic in embracing laparoscopic colectomy for treatment of malignant disease. Nevertheless, in patients with advanced disease, or those who have known metastasis, laparoscopic colectomy may have a role in management. The first access for laparoscopic colectomy is placed at the periumbilical area for introduction of the abdominal-wall lifter and the laparoscope. A small incision is then made for the mobilization of the colon. The incision is placed at access position no. 2 for right colectomy, no. 3 for transverse colectomy, no. 4 for left colectomy, and no. 5 for sigmoid colectomy (Figure 9.14). Swanstrom proposes other variations for the

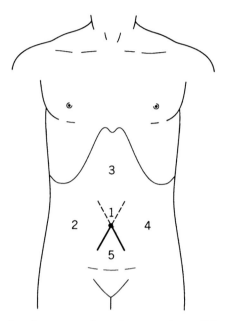

Figure 9.14. Diagram showing access for colectomy. A small incision is used for access as soon as diagnostic laparoscopy confirms the laparoscopic resectability of the colon lesion. The Laparofan® may need to be rotated several times during the procedure in order to facilitate the dissection.

use of these accesses and should be reviewed by the reader prior to embarking on gasless laparoscopic colectomy.[3] Five or six accesses may be needed for colectomy. One can easily use intra- or extracorporeal anastomotic technique for performing colon anastomosis. Conventional instruments as well as stapling devices are frequently used in the mobilization of the colon and in performing the anastomosis.

Colostomy

Laparoscopic colostomy is indicated for patients who have (1) advanced malignant disease causing bowel obstruction, (2) bowel control problem, and (3) colonic or rectal fistula that need a two-stage repair. Colostomy takedown with the gasless technique is indicated for malignant and nonmalignant diseases but may be especially favorable for trauma patients who have a diverting colostomy; by using laparoscopic techniques, a healthy trauma victim likely able to resume his or her activities sooner than one who has colostomy takedown by open technique.

A site on the abdomen is tattooed by the surgeon at the beginning of the procedure for colostomy stoma. After the first access is placed in the periumbilical position, a careful diagnostic laparoscopy is performed to examine the patient for adhesion. If necessary, an additional access can be placed in a diamond-shaped pattern for adhesiolysis. The skin and the full thickness of the abdominal wall are cored out as in conventional open colostomy placement (Figure 9.15). The colon is mobilized and exteriorized with Babcock clamps via this newly created abdominal-wall opening. End colostomy is performed with the use of a bowel stapler. The colostomy is anchored on the abdominal wall with nonabsorbable sutures. After closure of the remaining access, the colostomy is matured with absorbable suture (Figure 9.16).

Colostomy takedown uses similar accesses like those used in colostomy placement. After accesses are placed for diagnostic laparoscopy and adhesiolysis, the colostomy is freed from the abdominal wall and allowed to drop back into the abdominal cavity. The remaining opening on the abdominal wall becomes an extra excess allowing the surgeon to perform direct inspection of intraabdominal contents as well as digital examination of the bowels. Some-

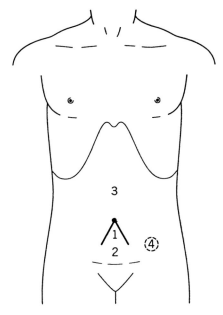

Figure 9.15. Access placement for sigmoid colostomy. Access 4 can be used for the mobilization of the sigmoid colon as well as for the placement of the sigmoid colostomy.

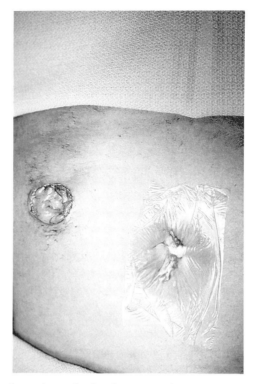

Figure 9.16. Picture of a patient who has laparoscopic sigmoid colostomy. (See insert for color representation.)

times, a flexible sigmoidoscope is inserted for identification and mobilization of the distal colonic stump (see Chapter 1). The anastomosis is done with a bowel stapler.

Derotation of Volvulus

Laparoscopic fixation of sigmoid volvulus has been reported by Miller and associates.[4] At UCD–East Bay, a similar technique has been used by Peskin and colleagues in treating a patient with pancreatic cancer and status post-Whipple procedure who presented with sigmoid volvulus.[5] In this patient, the first access was placed at the periumbilical area. A flexible sigmoidoscope was placed into the rectum to derotate the sigmoid volvulus and act as a "handle" in placing the bowel on the anterior abdominal wall. Two other accesses were placed on the abdominal wall as shown in Figure 9.17 for the surgeon to tack down the colon to the anterior abdominal wall with conventional silk sutures.

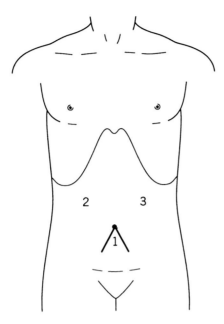

Figure 9.17. Access for sigmoidpexy.

IV. PELVIC PROCEDURES

Appendectomy

Laparoscopic appendectomy can be performed with three accesses (Figure 9.4). Although conventional instruments are used for most of the dissection, the appendix is usually transacted with an endoscopic stapler or in between two endoscopic ties at the base of the appendix. It is possible to use conventional suturing techniques for laparoscopic appendectomy but the larger size of the access required may take away some of the advantages of this minimally invasive technique. Copious amounts of irrigation and a pool-suction device are used to clean the right lower quadrant and pelvis.

Hernia Repair

The indication of laparoscopic herniorrhaphy is still controversial at this time; at UCD–East Bay, laparoscopic hernia repair is only used for selected patients. Indications for laparoscopic hernia repair include: (1) patients with bilateral hernias, (2) recurrent hernia, and (3) patients who are undergoing another con-

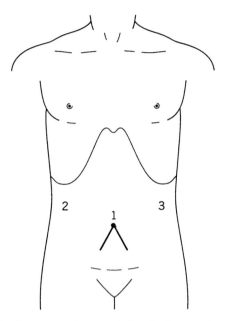

Figure 9.18. Access for laparoscopic transabdominal properitoneal herniorrhaphy.

comitant laparoscopic procedure. Figure 9.18 shows the accesses used for laparoscopic herniorrhaphy; the reader should note that the accesses are placed more laterally than with the conventional laparoscopic technique using pneumoperitoneum because of the partial obstruction caused by the abdominal-wall lifter. The author likes to use conventional instruments for the dissection (Figure 9.19). However, the mesh material used for the hernia repair is still secured with an endoscopic stapling device in order to minimize the size of the access. Besides the transabdominal–preperitoneal approach used by the author, Ferzli and Dysarz have used the complete extraperitoneal approach under epidural anesthesia for gasless laparoscopic herniorrhaphy.[6] With the continuous investigation of the planar lifting technique, it may one day be possible to use conventional sutures for performing gasless herniorrhaphy.

Peritoneal Dialysis Catheter Placement

Laparoscopic placement of a peritoneal dialysis (PD) catheter is indicated for patients who have had previous surgery or peritonitis, which may have resulted in intraabdominal adhesions. Laparoscopic management of the peritoneal

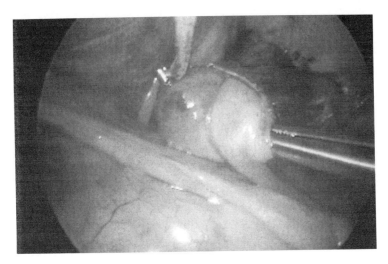

Figure 9.19. Cord structure is being isolated with a conventional right-angle clamp. (See insert for color representation.)

dialysis catheter is indicated for patients who have mechanical flow problems with the dialysis catheter. It is also used to perform laparoscopic biopsy of the peritoneum to rule out peritoneal fibrosis (Figure 9.20). Intravenous sedation and local anesthesia are employed for placement of the PD catheter unless the patient shows signs of intolerance. The first and perhaps the only access needed for the PD catheter placement is located at the periumbilical area. A 5-mm

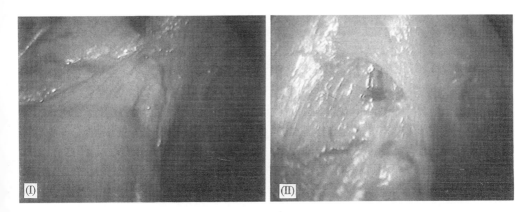

Figure 9.20. (I) A CAPD patient who has been diagnosed to have peritoneal fibrosis during laparoscopy. (II) Thick fibrous tissue was partially removed with endoscopic instruments. (See insert for color representation.)

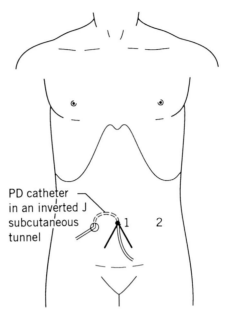

PD catheter
in an inverted J
subcutaneous
tunnel

Figure 9.21. Access for placement of peritoneal dialysis catheter.

endoscopic dissector or scissors can be placed in this access behind the laparoscope to manipulate the bowel or the PD catheter. If necessary, access numbers
2 and 3 at the paramedian area are used for introducing endoscopic instruments. In addition, the skin incision made for accesses 2 or 3 can be the exit site
of the external portion of the PD catheter. The author makes an inverted "J"-
shaped tunnel for the subcutaneous portion of the PD catheter to minimize
catheter tract infection (Figure 9.21). The peritoneum is closed with absorbable
sutures and 1500 cc of dialysate is infused into the abdomen to check catheter's
function and for possible leakage at the access site.

V. OTHER PROCEDURES

Gynecologic Procedures

The use of gasless laparoscopy appears to be growing more rapidly in gynecologic surgery. Since the first report by Hill and colleagues in using gasless lap-

aroscopy for hysterectomies, myomectomies, and ovarian cystectomies, the planar abdominal lifter has become the method of choice for some gynecologist in performing laparoscopic hysterectomy as well as for bladder-neck suspension in women with urinary incontinence.[7,8]

Lymph Nodes Biopsy for Stagging

The role of laparoscopic lymph-node staging for gynecologic or urilogic cancers is still controversial. Massaad and Ferzli have reported their experience of using the planar-lifting technique for pelvic lymph node dissection.[9] Like other surgeons who have reported their experiences with gasless techniques, the author also prefer to use conventional instruments to perform node sampling procedures (Figure 9.22a).

Vascular Procedures

One of the most exciting applications of the gasless technique is in aorto–femoral bypass surgery; since CO_2 pneumoperitoneum is not used for exposure, it is not necessary to operate in a sealed environment and therefore there is less risk of a gas embolus. Dion and associates successfully developed an animal model initially and subsequently in humans using the gasless retroperitoneal approach for aorto–femoral bypass.[10,11] Berens and Herde instead use a transabdominal approach for their aortic bypass procedures (Figure 9.22b).[12] All of these surgeons use conventional vascular surgical instruments and sutures for the anastomosis.

Spine Fusion Procedures

The use of a laparoscopic-assisted technique for exposure in spine fusion surgery and discectomy is still in the investigational stage. Multilevels discectomy and spine-fusion procedures can be performed with laparoscopic assisted techniques. The gasless technique adds a new dimension to this investigation by allowing spine surgeons to operate without concern of losing pneumoperitoneum (Figure 9.23).[13] Whether laparoscopic assisted spine surgery will replace conventional open technique is yet to be determined.

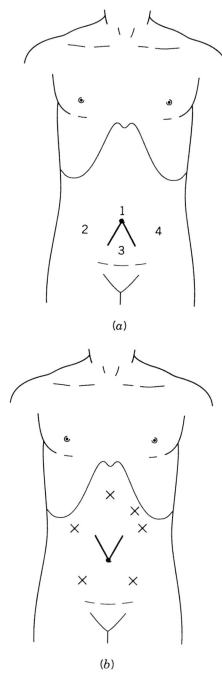

Figure 9.22. (*a*) Access for pelvic node dissection. (*b*) Access for aortic bypass surgery as suggested by Berens and Herde.[12]

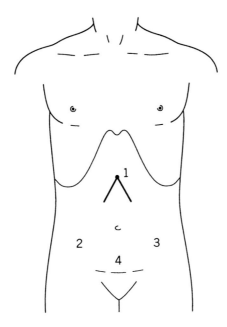

Figure 9.23. Access for laparoscopic L_5S_1 spine fusion. Access 4 is for placement of fusion cage or bone graft.

IV. CONCLUSION

Gasless laparoscopy with the planar lifter allows the surgeon to perform a variety of conventional procedures using minimally invasive techniques. The current available abdominal-wall lifters are still less than ideal since they obstruct the movements of the surgeon during the conduct of an operation. There is tremendous potential for the planar-lifting technique to become the gasless technique of choice over the wire-lifting system in view of the former's increasing popularity. Access into the abdomen using the planar-lifting system is easily obtained with miniincisions or trocars. The planar abdominal-wall lifting method will undoubtedly play an important role in the future development of gasless laparoscopic surgery.

REFERENCES

1. Tsoi EKM, Smith RS, Fry WR, et al.: "Laparoscopic surgery without pneumoperitoneum: A preliminary report." Surg Endosc 1993, 7:139 (Abstract).

2. Brams DM, Cardoza M, Smith RS: "Laparoscopic repair of traumatic gastric perforation using a gasless technique." J Laparoendosc Surg 1993, 3:587–591.

3. Swanstrom LL: "Gasless laparoscopic colectomy." In Smith RS and Organ CH (eds.), Gasless laparoscopy with conventional instruments. The next phase in minimally invasive surgery. San Francisco: Norman Publishing, 1993.

4. Miller R, Roe AM, Eltringham WK: "Laparoscopic fixation of sigmoid volvulus." Br J Surg 1992, 79:435.

5. Peskin G, Hirvela E, Tsoi EKM: unpublished data.

6. Ferzli GS, Dysarz FA: "Extraperitoneal inguinal herniorrhaphy performed without carbon dioxide insufflation." J Laparoendosc Surg 1994, 4:301–304.

7. Hill D, Maher P, Wood C, et al.: "Gasless laparoscopy." Aust NZ J Obstet Gynaecol 1994, 34:79–80.

8. Chin AK: personal communication.

9. Massaad A, Ferzli GS: "Gasless endoscopic extraperitoneal herniorrhaphy and pelvic node dissection." Surg Endosc 1994, 8–249 (Abstract).

10. Dion YM, Chin AK, Thompson TA: "Experimental laparoscopic aortobifemoral bypass." Surg Endosc 1995, 9:894–897.

11. Chin AK: personal communication.

12. Berens ES, Herde JR: "Laparoscopic vascular surgery: Four case reports." J Vasc Surg 1995, 22:73–79.

13. Tsoi EKM: unpublished data.

10

PROS AND CONS OF GASLESS LAPAROSCOPY

Edmund K. M. Tsoi, M.S., M.D.

I. INTRODUCTION

In Chapters 7–9, the development of the wire-lifting and planar-lifting techniques were reviewed in detail. In this chapter, the various advantages and disadvantages of gasless laparoscopy based on our experiences will be reviewed and shared with the reader.

II. PHYSIOLOGIC RESPONSE

The immediate advantage of the gasless technique is the lack of cardiopulmonary side effects from pneumoperitoneum (see Chapter 6). Low-pressure pneumoperitoneum (< 12 mm Hg) is an alternative for some patients who cannot tolerate standard pneumoperitoneum (15 mm Hg). There are those who will develop cardiovascular or pulmonary problems even at low pressure, i.e.,

Abdominal Access in Open and Laparoscopic Surgery
Edited by Edmund K. M. Tsoi and Claude H. Organ, Jr.
ISBN 0-471-13352-3 Copyright © 1996 by Wiley-Liss, Inc.

patients who have (1) hypovolemia, (2) severe cardiomyopathy, (3) severe pulmonary disease, (4) diaphragmatic hernia, and (5) selected trauma patients.

Rademaker and associates found that the planar abdominal-wall lifter did not alter the mean arterial pressure, central venous filling pressures, and cardiac output in eight pigs.[1] Woolley and colleagues found that when compared with pneumoperitoneum, the planar lifter causes significant reduction in central venous pressure, pulmonary capillary wedge pressure, and $PaCO_2$ in six adult domestic swine.[2] Furthermore, at above 10 cm H_2O PEEP, the experimental animals had a significantly lower cardiac index, system vascular index, and left ventricular stroke–work index than in the planar-lifter group.[2] Results of these two studies support the use of abdominal-wall lifter in cardiopulmonary compromised patients.

From our experience at the University of California, Davis (UCD)–East Bay Department of Surgery, we have observed that the exposure and the areas of abdominal wall proportionally elevated by the planar-lifting system in pigs are much larger than that of humans. Therefore, any physiological changes that is observed in pigs or other small experimental animals may not be applicable to humans. The planar abdominal-wall lifter or the wire-lifter function in essentially the same manner as conventional retractors used in open surgery (Richardson or Deaver retractors). As long as the mechanical abdominal-wall retractor does not compress the vena cava or other intraabdominal vessels, the physiological response should not be different than when using other retractors for pulling up the abdominal wall in open surgery. Another expected physiologic response seen in five pigs reported by Este-McDonald and associates is the lack of effect that the planar lifter has an intracranial pressure.[3] Again, the abdominal-wall retractor permits normal ventilation and therefore should not raise pCO_2 as does CO_2 pneumoperitoneum. Had we studied the physiologic responses of various mechanical retractors for open surgery in humans and compared them with the abdominal-wall lifters, the author speculates that they would be similar. An added advantage of the gasless system is its flexibility to convert to and from pneumoperitoneum for exposure if needed. However, if the operating room is not set up with the abdominal lifter prior to the beginning of the laparoscopic procedure, it is cumbersome and difficult to convert to the gasless technique. In this case, it may be wise for the surgeon to convert to open surgery or abort the procedure rather than insisting on pneumoperitoneum in the presence of undesirable physiologic responses.

III. SURGICAL TECHNIQUE

In Chapter 6, the authors have discussed the various complications associated with trocars used for traditional pneumoperitoneum laparoscopy. In our initial investigation with the planar-lifting system, we experienced one trocar-related small bowel injury that was promptly recognized and repaired.[4] Unlike pneumoperitoneum, the abdominal wall is maximally elevated at the point where there is lifter contact. Even at this point, the surgeon can still easily overcome the lifting force by using conventional laparoscopic trocars. Using miniincisions (< 1 cm) for access with or without the use of a blunt-tip trocar is not only safer but also reduces cost. If the miniincision is enlarged slightly by 2–3 cm, conventional open techniques can be used. The miniincision permits the surgeon to use conventional instruments for laparoscopic procedures; these instruments are sturdier than specialized laparoscopic instruments and more familiar to the surgeon. The use of high-volume irrigation and suction in maintaining a clear operating field is possible. Costs are further reduced by not using expensive specialized laparoscopic instruments.[5] Table 1 contains a list of instruments that are being used by us in performing gasless laparoscopic surgery.

Another advantage of using a small incision for access is that it allows the surgeon to perform direct visual inspection and digital examination of intraabdominal contents. Although laparoscopic ultrasound and three-dimensional video laparoscope can provide the surgeon with the customary "feel" of open surgery, there is still no effective substitute for the surgeon's tactile exam-

TABLE 10.1

Conventional instruments used in gasless laparoscopic surgery

Abdominal "fish" retractor	Metzenbaum scissors
Allis clamp	Needle driver
Army–Navy retractor	Pean clamp
Babcock clamp	Peanut dissector
Cholangiogram catheter	Pool suction device
Choledochoscope	Right angle clamp
Electrocautery	Sponge sticks
Kocher clamp	Stapling devices
Malleable retractor	Tonsil clamp

ination of the pathology. Furthermore, direct visual inspection is still superior than looking at a two-dimensional video screen. We call the direct inspection technique the "Laparo-look."

IV. CONTAMINATION RISKS

Gasless laparoscopic surgery has combined open and minimally invasive surgery by allowing the surgeon to operate in a semisealed environment without the fear of losing pneumoperitoneum. This semisealed environment becomes a barrier against the spreading of infectious material from the patient to the operating team. Eubanks and colleagues as well as Baggish have studied sprayback of body fluid that escapes the abdomen when pneumoperitoneum is accidentally released via the trocar.[6,7] With the gasless technique, the operating field is in an isobaric condition with the outside, since maintenance of intraabdominal CO_2 pressure for exposure is not needed. Therefore, the chances of being splashed by intraabdominal fluid are less than in open or traditional laparoscopic surgery. The author routinely places a pool-suction device into the abdomen to remove body fluids. Intraabdominal smoke generated by the cautery can also be evacuated via the trocar gas port or pool suction and consequently further lowers the exposure risk to the operating team, even when the patient has a known infectious disease such as HIV or hepatitis.

For the patient undergoing laparoscopic surgery with CO_2 pneumoperitoneum, there is the risk of spreading an isolated infectious process from one part of the abdomen to another. Concerns have been raised about reports of tumor spreading in the abdominal-wall port implants as well as within the abdomen soon after a conventional laparoscopic operation.[8,9] It is not clear whether the spreading of infectious material or tumor cells is caused by the CO_2 gas spray or because of direct contact by the disease process. Because the operating environment is isobaric, with the gasless technique, the gas-spreading theory is readily eliminated. In addition, the author routinely uses a large volume of irrigation in infectious cases to remove the contaminants; a long-term study will be needed to determine whether the gasless techniques will result in less contamination by infectious material or tumor cells.

V. SURGEONS' EDUCATION

One of the first observations the surgeon immediately notices when using the gasless technique is the difference in the exposure of the operating field this technique provides when compared with conventional laparoscopy using pneumoperitoneum. The tight, round, dome shape of the abdomen experienced with pneumoperitoneum is replaced by a trapezoid-shaped abdomen. The use of a lesser force for sharp trocar placement is recommended for surgeons who choose to not use miniincisions or blunt trocars for access.

Intraabdominal exposure is also different than that of pneumoperitoneum because its contents are not being "pushed aside" by the CO_2. Exposure of the lumber gutters are less than adequate unless a mechanical retractor is used for bowel retraction. One usually does not think that CO_2 can act as a bowel retractor, but when the abdomen is insufflated with CO_2, the diaphragm is elevated, creating extra space for the intraabdominal contents. The diaphragm is partially paralyzed unless the force of positive ventilation is great enough to push the diaphragm back into the abdomen and thus reduce this extra space. The force required to ventilate the patient will increase the peak airway pressure, and may result in barotrauma. Patients with underlying pulmonary disease will be especially susceptible. Using the gasless technique, the diaphragm is free to move with the respiratory cycle as in open surgery. Therefore the abdominal contents are frequently shifting unless mechanical retraction is applied. There are two ways to overcome the diaphragmatic movements related to shifting of abdominal contents without using retractors: (1) by shifting the patient's position so that gravitational force can help to pull the bowel away from the operating field; and (2) by requesting the anesthesiologist to use a smaller tidal volume with an increased respiratory rate to ventilate the patient. This latter maneuver will allow the anesthesiologist to ventilate the patient with the same minute volume and decrease the shifting of abdominal contents associated with diaphragmatic movements.

The learning curve for the surgeon is about 10 cases to become comfortable with gasless laparoscopy. Patient selection is an important determinant in deciding the success or failure of the initial procedures. After performing a variety of cases, I find that the ideal patient is one who is not excessively obese, with some laxity of the anterior abdominal wall. Access placement is also important in deciding the outcome of an operation with gasless laparoscopy. Whether one uses the wire lifter or the planar retractor, the abdominal-wall lifter will physically hinder the movements of surgical instruments inside the abdominal cavity. The accesses used by surgeons in conventional laparoscopy need to be modified to avoid "bumping" into the abdominal-wall retractor during dissection.

Once the surgeon becomes acclimated to the exposure, it is quite easy to adapt open techniques to gasless laparoscopy. In addition to the flexibility of using conventional instruments, local anesthesia together with intravenous sedation have been employed for selected procedures like diagnostic laparoscopy, gastrostomy, and peritoneal dialysis catheter placement. Ferzli and Dysarz have used epidural anesthesia to perform gasless extraperitoneal laparoscopic hernia repair in five patients.[10]

VI. CONCLUSION

Gasless laparoscopy appears to offer technical and physiological advantages over conventional laparoscopy with CO_2 pneumoperitoneum for exposure. The gasless technique reduces the operating team exposure to infectious patient contamination because the operating field is semienclosed and high-volume suction can be used to evacuate body fluids and vaporized tissues. The access into the abdomen is easy to obtain because the surgeon can use trocars or incisions and need not worry about the necessity of maintaining a sealed operating environment. Conventional instruments can be used and lessons one learned in open surgery can be easily adapted to the gasless technique. The learning curve for surgeons will vary until they become acclimated to the shifting abdominal contents associated with diaphragmatic movements and the hinderance caused by the abdominal-wall retractor. Once the surgeon overcomes the bias from previous experience with pneumoperitoneum for exposure, no special training or weekend courses are needed to use the planar lifter. The gasless technique appears to be the missing link between traditional access by incision in open surgery and conventional laparoscopic access by trocar and pneumoperitoneum. Gasless laparoscopy should be added to the armamentarium of access techniques for surgeons interested in minimally invasive surgery.

REFERENCES

1. Rademaker BMP, Meyer DW, Bannenberg JJG, et al.: "Laparoscopy without pneumoperitoneum. Effects of abdominal wall retraction versus carbon dioxide insufflation on hemodynamics and gas exchange in pigs." Surg Endosc 1995, 9:797–801.

2. Woolley DS, Puglisi RN, Bilgrami S, et al.: "Comparison of the hemodynamic effects of gasless abdominal distention and CO_2 pneumoperitoneum during incremental positive end-expiratory pressure." J Surg Res 1995, 58:75–80.

3. Este-McDonald JR, Josephs LG, Birkett DH, et al.: "Changes in intracranial pressure associated with apneumic retractors." Arch Surg 1995, 130:362–366.

4. Tsoi EKM, Smith RS, Fry WR, et al.: "Laparoscopic surgery without pneumoperitoneum: A preliminary report." Surg Endosc 1993, 7:139 (abstract).

5. Smith RS, Fry WR, Tsoi EKM, et al.: "Gasless laparoscopy with conventional instruments: The next phase in minimally invasive surgery." Arch Surg 1993, 128:1102–1107.

6. Eubanks S, Newman L, Lucas G: "Reduction of HIV transmission during laparoscopic procedures." Surg Laparosc Endosc 1993, 3:2–5.

7. Baggish MS: "Comparison of smoke and sprayback leakage from two different trocar sleeves during operative laparoscopy." J Gynecol Surg 1993, 9:65–76.

8. Ramos JM, Gupta S, Anthone GJ, et al.: "Laparoscopy and colon cancer. Is the port site at risk? A preliminary report." Arch Surg 1994, 129:897–900.

9. Cirocco WC, Schwartzman A, Golub RW: "Abdominal wall recurrence after laparoscopic colectomy for colon cancer." Surgery 1994, 116:842–846.

10. Ferzli GS, Dysarz FA: "Extraperitoneal endoscopic inguinal herniorrhaphy performed without carbon dioxide insufflation." J Laparoendosc Surg 1994, 4:301–304.

11

FUTURE CONSIDERATIONS

Edmund K. M. Tsoi, M.S., M.D.
Claude H. Organ, Jr., M.D.

I. INTRODUCTION

The authors have discussed how surgical access to the abdominal contents has changed from the use of traditional incisions to trocars and miniincisions. The driving force behind the scene that enables these changes is the development of complex miniature integrated circuits (ICs). The small video camera used in videoscopic surgery is the prime example of a device built from ICs. In this chapter, we will discuss new developments in laparoscopic-assisted techniques and other electronic devices that may change the future of abdominal surgical access.

II. NEW ACCESS TECHNIQUES FOR OPEN SURGERY

One of the difficulties encountered by surgeons using gasless techniques is the current limitations of surgical instrument movements caused by the abdomi-

Abdominal Access in Open and Laparoscopic Surgery
Edited by Edmund K. M. Tsoi and Claude H. Organ, Jr.
ISBN 0-471-13352-3 Copyright © 1996 by Wiley-Liss, Inc.

nal-wall lifter. As more experience is gained with gasless laparoscopy at the University of California, Davis (UCD)–East Bay Department of Surgery, video laparoscopic techniques are applied to open surgery as the continued study of the abdominal-wall lifter evolves. The use of miniincisions in advanced laparoscopic surgery has given us the opportunity of combining incisions as a substitute for laparoscopic access into the abdomen. In the future, the magnifying power of the lens and light source attached to the laparoscope will enable visualization of the intraabdominal and intrathoracic structures via a small-access open surgery, thereby avoiding problems associated with a conventional incision in open surgery or with pneumoperitoneum in laparoscopic surgery. Another way to view this development is to conceptualize it as gasless laparoscopic surgery without using wires or a lifter for exposure. As an example, in the beginning of an exploratory laparotomy, a small incision is made to allow the placement of a small retractor (Army–Navy or Richardson retractor) and a video laparoscope. From the video picture, we can obtain additional information in guiding our incision, and may even obtain enough information in the diagnosis and treatment to avoid an extended incision (Figure 11.1).

Video-assisted open laparoscopy is similar to the technique proposed by Tyagi and colleagues in using the video laparoscope to perform open cholecystectomy at the "minimal stress triangle."[1] A variation of the open videoscopic-assisted technique has been proposed by Kusminsky and associates for staging laparotomy. They make a small incision for placement of the

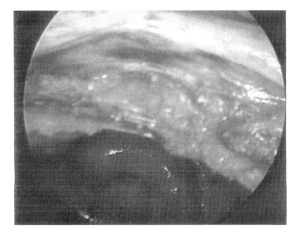

Figure 11.1. A small incision is made for placement of an Army–Navy retractor and a video-laparoscope at the beginning of exploratory laparotomy. (See insert for color representation.)

assistant surgeon's hand for bowel manipulation and pneumoperitoneum for exposure.[2]

Another variation of open endoscopically assisted surgery that has shown great promise is in mediastinal surgery. We have performed videoscopic-assisted ileal interposition for esophageal replacement, and others have performed transhiatal esophagectomy with gastric-tube interposition.[3,4] Yim and Ho have recommended a miniincision in the subxiphoid area to perform videoscopic-assisted subxiphoid pericardiotomy.[5]

In view of the development of these new access techniques to the mediastinum and upper abdominal structures, in the future, procedures such as biliary and pancreatic surgery, antireflux procedures, and antiulcer surgery will be performed in increasing numbers with videoscopic-assisted open techniques via a miniincision without pneumoperitoneum or an abdominal-wall lifter. The key to the development of such techniques is an understanding of abdominal and thoracic body-wall dynamics, which allows the surgeon to find areas in these cavities with properties similar to those of the "minimal stress triangle."[1]

Chapter 10 delineates the advantages of the gasless laparoscopic technique combined with the ability in utilizing conventional instruments (e.g., right-angle clamp, abdominal pool-suction device, needle holder, peanut dissector, babcock clamp, gastrointestinal stapling devices etc.). Conventional extralong surgical instruments are adequate for gasless procedures when the distance between the pivot point of the instrument is far enough from the tip and allows the surgeon to open and close the jaws freely with a greater circumference expansion. Nagai (Chapter 8) discusses modifications to increase the flexibility of conventional surgical instruments. We have used thoracoscopic instruments in cases without pneumoperitoneum, but the results are far from ideal. With increased attention to cost reduction in health care, surgical-instrument companies should redesign conventional instruments to better facilitate open and gasless laparoscopic procedures. With increasing interest in videoscopic-assisted open surgery, such modified conventional instruments will definitely play a vital role in the development of this access technique.

III. NEW IMAGING TECHNIQUES

The most sophisticated device built with ICs is the computer. Computers currently available can generate lifelike images that mimic reality. To date, virtual-reality simulation of the interior of body is in an early stage of development. Improved virtual-reality technology will be able to create three-dimensional images and replace the use of the conventional dual-camera technique. Begin and colleagues have recently reported their initial results with robotic technology in laparoscopic surgery.[6] A flexible, robotic camera together with the use of virtual-reality technology will enable surgeons to utilize smaller access into the abdomen or thorax and simultaneously permit immediate consultation with colleagues in other parts of the country who are interconnected via these computer terminals. Together with intraoperative ultrasound and/or intraoperative contrast studies (dye or fluorescein), imaging technology will certainly be able to guide the surgeon to the pathology through minimally invasive access.[7-9] Critics may still say "seeing" is not enough: an adequate access into the body cavity must also allow the surgeon to touch the pathology. Recently, Ohtsuka and colleagues reported the development of a tactile sensor that enables them to detect lung tumors in thoracoscopic surgery.[10] Such technology in the future will be expanded and surgeons will utilize computerized sensors to identify various intraabdominal pathology regardless of the access technique.

IV. CONCLUSION

The future of surgical access into the abdomen in open and laparoscopic surgery continues to evolve with new developments in science and technology. The revolution from traditional long incisions for access into the peritoneal cavity to a combination of trocars and miniincisions continues to evolve. The development of gasless techniques for exposure, and the creative use videolaparoscopy in open surgery demonstrates that surgeons continue to combine their innovative ideas with technology to improve the techniques of surgical access into the abdomen. Yet the fundamental principles of surgery will not change regardless of how the access is obtained. An access must allow surgeons to obtain adequate exposure to perform a procedure safely.

REFERENCES

1. Tyagi NS, Meredith MC, Lumb JC, et al.: "A new minimally invasive technique for cholecystectomy: subxiphoid 'minimal stress triangle' microceliotomy." Ann Surg 1994, 220:617–525.

2. Kusminsky RE, Tiley EH, Lucente FC, et al.: "Laparoscopic staging laparotomy with intra-abdominal manipulation." Surg Laparosc Endosc 1994, 4:103–105.

3. Tsoi EKM, Harness JK: unpublished data.

4. Sadanaga N, Kuwano H, Watanabe M, et al.: "Laparoscopy-assisted surgery: A new technique for transhiatal esophageal dissection." Am J Surg 1994, 168:355–357.

5. Yim APC, Ho JKS: "Video-assisted subxiphoid pericardiectomy." J Laparoendosc Surg 1995, 5:193–198.

6. Begin E, Gagner M, Hurteau R, et al.: "A robotic camera for laparoscopic surgery: Conception and experimental results." Surg Laparosc Endosc 1995, 1:6–11.

7. John TG, Grieg JD, Crosbie JL, et al.: "Superior staging of liver tumors with laparoscopy and laparoscopic ultrasound." Ann Surg 1994, 220:711–719.

8. Kam DM, Scheeres DE: "Fluorescein-assisted laparoscopy in the identification of arterial mesenteric ischemia." Surg Endosc 1993, 7:75–78.

9. Edye M, Schwartz M, Miller C: "Preoperative laparoscopic portal venography and endoluminal biopsy streamlines liver transplantation protocol for hepatocellular carcinoma." Surg Endosc 1994, 8–973 (Abstract).

10. Ohtsuka T, Konno T, Nakajima J: "New Tactile sensor for detecting the lung tumor in thoracoscopic surgery." Surg Endosc 1994, 8–1013 (Abstract).

INDEX